THE **COMPACT C**

Series Editor: Yvonne D Arcy, MS, CRNP, CNS

Compact Clinical Guide to
CHRONIC PAIN MANAGEMENT:
An Evidence-Based Approach for Nurses
Yvonne D'Arcy, MS, CRNP, CNS

Compact Clinical Guide to
ACUTE PAIN MANAGEMENT:
An Evidence-Based Approach for Nurses
Yvonne D'Arcy, MS, CRNP, CNS

Compact Clinical Guide to
CRITICAL CARE, TRAUMA AND EMERGENCY
PAIN MANAGEMENT:
An Evidence-Based Approach for Nurses
Liza Marmo, MSN, RN, CCRN

Compact Clinical Guide to
GERIATRIC PAIN MANAGEMENT:
An Evidence-Based Approach for Nurses
Ann Quinlan-Colwell, PhD, RNC, AHNBC, FAAPM

Compact Clinical Guide to
INFANT AND CHILD PAIN MANAGEMENT:
An Evidence-Based Approach for Nurses
Linda L. Oakes, MSN, RN-BC, CCNS

Yvonne D'Arcy, MS, CRNP, CNS, is an expert pain management and palliative care nurse practitioner who has received several awards for nursing excellence, and who possesses a remarkable publishing and presentation career history. Currently, Ms. D'Arcy is the nurse practitioner for Pain Management and Palliative Care at Suburban Hospital–Johns Hopkins Medicine, in Bethesda, Maryland. She has significant experience in pain management, having worked as Oncology Pain Service and Staff Education Coordinator at Johns Hopkins Oncology Center; Acute Pain Service Coordinator and Pain Clinic Supervisor at the Mayo Clinic in Jacksonville, Florida; and Pain Center Manager and Clinical Coordinator of the Acute Pain Service at the Heartland Health System in St. Joseph, Missouri. Her accomplishments include delivering more than 100 poster and oral presentations, publishing more than 100 journal articles on pain-related topics, authoring 3 books on pain, serving as a consultant for hospitals and health care providers, providing peer review for and serving on the editorial boards of *Nursing, The Journal for Nurse Practitioners*, and *Pain Management News*. Ms. D'Arcy has been an active member of the American Society of Pain Management Nurses, having served on the Board of Directors and as Chairman of the Clinical Practice Committee, is a member of the American Pain Society, and serves as a member of the Clinical Guidelines Committee and the American Academy of Nurse Practitioners. She is the recipient of the Nursing Spectrum Excellence Division Award for Advancing and Leading the Profession.

Compact Clinical Guide to

CHRONIC PAIN MANAGEMENT

An Evidence-Based Approach for Nurses

Yvonne D'Arcy, MS, CRNP, CNS

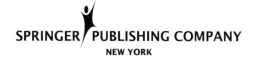

SPRINGER PUBLISHING COMPANY
NEW YORK

Copyright © 2011 Springer Publishing Company, LLC
All rights reserved.

No part of this publication may be reproduced, stored in a retrieval system, or transmitted in any form or by any means, electronic, mechanical, photocopying, recording, or otherwise, without the prior permission of Springer Publishing Company, LLC, or authorization through payment of the appropriate fees to the Copyright Clearance Center, Inc., 222 Rosewood Drive, Danvers, MA 01923, 978-750-8400; fax 978-646-8600, info@copyright.com or on the web at www.copyright.com.

Springer Publishing Company, LLC
11 West 42nd Street
New York, NY 10036
www.springerpub.com

Acquisitions Editor: Margaret Zuccarini
Senior Editor: Rose Mary Piscitelli
Cover design: Steven Pisano
Composition: Absolute Service, Inc./Pablo Apostol, Project Manager

ISBN: 978-0-8261-0540-0
E-book ISBN: 978-0-8261-0548-6

11   12   13   5   4   3   2   1

The author and the publisher of this Work have made every effort to use sources believed to be reliable to provide information that is accurate and compatible with the standards generally accepted at the time of publication. Because medical science is continually advancing, our knowledge base continues to expand. Therefore, as new information becomes available, changes in procedures become necessary. We recommend that the reader always consult current research and specific institutional policies before performing any clinical procedure. The author and publisher shall not be liable for any special, consequential, or exemplary damages resulting in whole or in part from the readers' use of or reliance on the information contained in this book. The publisher has no responsibility for the persistence or accuracy of URLs for external or third-party Internet websites referred to in this publication and does not guarantee that any content on such websites is or will remain accurate or appropriate.

Library of Congress Cataloging-in-Publication Data
D'Arcy, Yvonne M.
  Compact clinical guide to chronic pain management : an evidence-based approach / Yvonne D'Arcy.
    p. ; cm.
  Includes bibliographical references.
  ISBN 978-0-8261-0540-0 (alk. paper)— ISBN 978-0-8261-0548-6 (e-book)
  1. Chronic pain—Treatment—Handbooks, manuals, etc.   I. Title.
  [DNLM: 1. Pain—drug therapy.   2. Pain—nursing.
  3. Analgesics—therapeutic use.   4. Chronic Disease—drug therapy.
  5. Evidence-Based Nursing.   6. Primary Health Care. WY 160.5]
  RB127.D378 2011
  616'.0472—dc22
                                              2010032175

Special discounts on bulk quantities of our books are available to corporations, professional associations, pharmaceutical companies, health care organizations, and other qualifying groups.
If you are interested in a custom book, including chapters from more than one of our titles, we can provide that service as well. **For details, please contact:**
Special Sales Department, Springer Publishing Company, LLC
11 West 42nd Street, 15th Floor, New York, NY 10036-8002
Phone: 877-687-7476 or 212-431-4370; Fax: 212-941-7842
Email: sales@springerpub.com

Printed in the United States of America by Hamilton Printing

*This book is dedicated to all the practitioners
who work with patients who have chronic pain of all types.
These patients are a group of special people with individual
needs and hopes. For all the hard work, time, and
dedication you have extended to these patients,
I express my sincere appreciation.*

Contents

Foreword

Nurse practitioners (NPs) are the fastest growing group of practitioners in primary care practice. There are currently 125,000 NPs who are licensed to practice, with the majority working in primary care. In 2008, 8,000 NPs graduated from NP educational programs. Growth-wise, the current U.S. Government Accountability Office report on growth and trends in primary care indicates that primary care NPs are increasing at a rate of 9.44% per capita compared with 1.77% per capita for medical doctors in primary care.

Simultaneously, the number of aging Americans has steadily increased with the entry of the baby boomers into the ranks of those patients who are candidates for chronic pain complaints, such as osteoarthritis, low back pain, and other degenerative pain conditions. In primary care, pain is one of the biggest reasons that patients seek help from health care providers. About 26 million people in the United States suffer from severe pain at least monthly. In the working population, pain is responsible for one-fourth of all sick time lost from work, or 50 million lost workdays per year. Unfortunately, about 28% of Americans with pain do not feel that there is any real solution for their pain.

Research in pain management is trying to provide new solutions and answers to these difficult-to-treat patients who have complex pain needs. There are many new guidelines and position statements, both general and disease-specific, that make practice recommendations for using long-term opioid therapy, diagnosing and treating low back pain, and use of medication such as methadone. Genetic factors are being studied to determine which patients have the best outcomes with certain pain medications. New technology is grow-ing every day so that new delivery systems are available to deliver the available pain medications.

This book is a comprehensive guide to treating chronic pain. NPs will find information on prescribing opioids safely, pain assess-ment, and interventional options for pain relief. Using opioid agree-ments, performing urine screens, and learning to screen patients for potential problems when opioids are initiated are all detailed, with examples of screening tools and agreements.

The author is an NP who sees many patients with chronic pain in her practice. She has many years of experience diagnosing and treating patients with chronic pain, and she is considered to be a leader in her field. She is sharing her expertise and experiences in this book so that other NPs can provide high-quality pain management to their patients and get positive outcomes. The book provides easy-to-use features and case studies, and will be a useful addition to any clinician's references for clinical practice.

Bill McCarberg, MD
Founder, Chronic Pain Management Program
Kaiser Permanente
San Diego, California

I

Overview and Assessment of Chronic Pain

1

The Problem of Chronic Pain

INTRODUCTION TO CHRONIC, PERSISTENT PAIN

Health care providers are seeing larger numbers of patients with chronic, persistent pain than ever before. The causes of the pain are varied, but they all still have the potential for disability, decreased functionality, and decreased quality of life. The number of patients with chronic pain has increased nationally to the point that many health care providers consider chronic pain to be a major national public health problem (Trescot et al., 2008).

What we do know about most nurse practitioners is that they feel that their basic nurse practitioner education did not prepare them to treat patients with chronic pain. In a survey of 400 nurse practitioners, 62% of the respondents felt they had been prepared to assess patients with chronic pain, whereas 38% indicated they did not feel prepared. When treatment of chronic pain was queried, only 44% of the respondents felt they had been prepared to treat chronic pain, whereas 56% felt they had not been prepared (D'Arcy, 2009a). When asked to choose which of the concerns were most important when prescribing opioids for chronic pain, the same survey group indicated the following concerns from most important to least important:

1. Cost
2. Fear of regulatory oversight

3. Addiction
4. Not knowledgeable enough about medications
5. Don't want to be seen as different from other prescribers (D'Arcy, 2009a)

These fears of regulatory oversight and legal consequences are also colored by fears of addicting patients to opioids when long-term opioid therapy is used to treat chronic pain. When the survey respondents were asked how comfortable they were with prescribing opioids for 12 months or more when the patient had chronic pain, only one third of the respondents felt they had a good comfort level with the practice (D'Arcy, 2009a). These findings are consistent with those of other surveys on pain management knowledge and attitudes that have been used for several years.

Despite national efforts to teach patients and prescribers about chronic pain by declaring 2000 to 2010 as the Decade of Pain Control and Research, we have made little headway. Moreover, pain is still undertreated. Although only approximately 5% of patients in primary care develop a substance abuse disorder/addiction with long-term opioid use, including all of those patients who have been exposed to opioids and those patients who had never used opioids, these outdated perceptions still persist (Fishbain, Cole, Lewis, Rosomoff, & Rosomoff, 2008). Although there are other studies that categorize substance abuse disorders and opioid misuse differently and have different statistical findings, the endpoint is that true addiction is not as common as prescribers perceive it to be, and most patients with chronic pain can tolerate long-term opioid therapy successfully.

Who are these patients with chronic pain and what are their complaints? Because chronic, persistent pain is now considered a chronic illness, how can these patients cope with the long-term nature of the condition? What types of treatments are available? What is the best way to assess pain in these patients? The following chapters of this book will answer these questions and provide evidence-based information on many aspects of chronic, persistent pain.

PREVALENCE OF CHRONIC PAIN

A patient with chronic pain may be anyone you see or know. They may be young or old, wealthy or homeless. Chronic pain does not respect age, race, financial status, or gender. It can affect anyone at any time, and the effects of the pain can be life changing. The pain can be the result of surgery, an injury, disease, or treatments such as chemotherapy, or it may just start for no apparent reason. Once the pain occurs, it will affect every aspect of the person's life. Every patient with chronic pain has a story to tell of how the pain has changed their lives and how they have learned to adapt and cope with it.

Chronic, persistent pain accounts for 40 million patient visits annually and is the most common reason that patients seek help from health care professionals. On average, chronic pain patient has:

- Had pain for 7 years
- Had three major surgeries
- Incurred medical bills of $50,000 to $100,000

There are many different types of chronic pain. Responses to a survey by Research America indicate that the most common types of chronic pain include the following:

- Back pain (28%)
- Arthritis and joint pain (19%)
- Headaches/migraine (17%)
- Knee pain (17%)
- Shoulder pain (7%)

Low back pain, the most common type of chronic pain, has become a common complaint in the American health care system. The normal aging process causes the spinal discs to desiccate and flatten. By age 20, the vascularity of the spinal discs decreases and by age 30, the desiccation of the disc can cause fissures to develop in the endplates of the vertebral bodies (D'Arcy, 2009). Because of these spinal changes that occur as we age, it is estimated that 95% of the population will have the beginning of degenerative disc disease by age 50 (D'Arcy, 2009b). Patients who are at risk for low back pain, the most common type of chronic pain, include the following:

- Those who are older than 55 years
- Obese patients
- Those with poor physical condition and who do not engage in regular exercise
- Lower socioeconomic groups who have fewer opportunities to access health care
- Workers who have engaged in heavy labor over time
- Those with reduced spinal canal dimensions (spinal stenosis) (D'Arcy, 2009b)

Unfortunately, the picture of chronic pain for the older patients is even more grim. The American Geriatrics Society estimates that 80% of patients in long-term care facilities experience chronic daily pain. Assessing and treating pain in these patients is difficult because of the high incidence of dementia and nonverbal patients. The story for community-dwelling elders is a little better, with 25% to 50% of them reporting chronic pain that affects their ability to function. No matter what the age of the patient with chronic pain is, there is an impact on the way these patients lead their lives.

COSTS OF CHRONIC PAIN

The cost of chronic, persistent pain cannot be fully measured, because it includes not only lost work time, or increased health care utilization, but also personal and quality-of-life issues, which have costs that cannot be calculated. Patients with chronic pain are often misunderstood and undertreated for the pain. As they seek relief for their pain, the health care system may view them as drug seeking rather than relief seeking. This may cause the chronic pain patient to present a social mask to the public that hides the full extent of the pain. Assessing pain in a patient who is trying to hide the effects of chronic pain is much more difficult and requires a comprehensive set of questions to obtain the needed information.

Most patients with chronic pain report pain that exists at some level throughout the day. The patients with low back pain may have episodes of pain in which the pain increases and then returns to a lower, more tolerable level. Along with the pain, patients can become anxious or depressed as the pain appears to be untreatable or as pain intensity increases. The uncertainty of the pain experience can lead patients to feel helpless and hopeless.

Monetary Costs

It is difficult to measure the cost of chronic pain. The best evaluation is that chronic pain costs are estimated to be $100 billion per year and are related to the following:

- Health care
- Welfare and disability costs
- Losses in tax revenue
- Lost productivity through both absenteeism and presentism (at work, but in pain)

Presentism alone is estimated to cost $61.2 billion per year (Stewart, Ricci, Chee, Morganstein, & Lipton, 2003). Most patients with chronic pain want to work but are limited by pain. Because these patients try to work but are less productive, it is a hidden cost that is hard to evaluate.

Personal Costs

Pain that is long term can take a toll on money and employment, but it can also rob the patient of quality of life, disrupt sleep, and cause significant depression. Depression is a common occurrence in patients with chronic pain. The depression is more of a situational depression than a deep-seated clinical effect. If depression is a part of a patient's chronic pain, treatment with antidepressants is indicated. If the depression is allowed to go untreated, the patient may develop suicidal ideation. Unfortunately, the rate for suicide in chronic pain patients is twice the rate for the similar patient demographic without chronic pain (Tang & Crane, 2006).

Chronic pain can also result in sleep disturbances, which can rob the patients of needed rest and restorative sleep they need to help them cope with the stress of daily life with pain. Sleep disturbances are common and occurred in about 55% of patients in one study who reported restless/or light sleep after the onset of pain (Marin, Cyhan, & Miklos, 2006). The most common adverse effects of sleep disturbances that are reported by patients include the following:

- Delayed onset of sleep
- Daytime fatigue
- Nonrestorative sleep

The personal costs for the older patient with chronic pain are very significant. Because prescribers are reluctant to provide high-level opioid medications to many older patients, for fear of unwanted side effects such as oversedation, constipation, and confusion, the pain will be untreated or undertreated (Bruckenthal & D'Arcy, 2007). Undertreated pain can lead to the following:

- Depression, anxiety
- Decreased socialization
- Sleep disturbances
- Impaired ambulation and functioning
- Increased health care utilization and costs (Bruckenthal & D'Arcy, 2007)

Chronic pain can lead to poor self-esteem, financial ruin, and diminished quality of life. It affects the health status of the patient by suppressing natural killer cells, decreasing the body's ability to defend itself against tumor and virus-infected cells. Chronic pain not only reduces the quality of life but also can have an impact on life itself.

PAIN TRANSMISSION

Pain Theories

The mechanisms of pain transmission are different for acute pain and chronic pain. The onset of acute pain is sudden and can provoke a fight or flight type of response, with adrenaline release that will subside rapidly. Chronic pain, on the other hand, is long term, and over time, more complex and advanced pain-facilitating responses, such as the activation of N-methyl-D-aspartate (NMDA) receptors, take place. Many pharmaceutical companies aim the action of their medications at a specific sites in the pain transmission process. As one example, retaining serotonin at the synaptic junction can help reduce the amount of pain-facilitating substances available to create or continue the pain stimulus.

There are theories that have been advanced over the years about how pain is transmitted and what physiologic mechanisms are involved. One of the earliest theorists was René Descartes who felt that pain was a stimulus response mechanism. This concept was also called the labeled line theory. In this theory, pain was seen as a painful stimulus that traveled up to the brain, resulting in the body recognizing the sensation as pain. An example would be a stimulus, such as a burn or trauma, that would travel up to the brain, and the brain would recognize it as pain. The resulting response would be for the body to withdraw from the pain, such as removing the hand from a fire. This theory focuses primarily on the physical aspect of pain rather than including the emotional or psychological aspects of the pain experience.

Especially for patients with chronic pain, the psychological and emotional component of pain is an important aspect of the condition. Older theories, such as those espoused by Pavlov, considered pain to be a learned response that was affected by cultural and learned behaviors that could be offset by operant conditioning. Turk described pain as a multidimensional experience and proposes that the patient, not the health care practitioner, is really the specialist on the pain. This theory empowers the patient to become active participants in pain treatment and helps the patient diminish negative behaviors and increase positive reinforcing behaviors (American Society for Pain Management Nursing [ASPMN], 2010).

Perhaps the most well known theory of pain transmission is the Gate Control Theory developed by Melzack and Wall in 1965 (ASPMN, 2010). In this theory, the psychological and physiological aspects of pain transmission are combined. Simplistically, the Gate Control Theory states that a pain stimulus can be significant enough in intensity to "open" a neuronal gate that will allow the pain stimulus to proceed up the nervous system to create a sensation that can be identified as pain by the brain.

The actual steps in pain transmission according to the Gate Control Theory include the following:

- A pain stimulus from the body periphery is carried by A-delta and C nerve fibers to the dorsal horn of the spinal cord.
- The gate is located in the substantia gelatinosa in the dorsal horn of the spinal cord, and it can facilitate or inhibit, either promote or stop, the progression of the nerve impulse through the central nervous system.
- If the painful stimulus is of sufficient intensity or persists, the pain is transmitted up through the limbic system to the cerebral cortex.
- In the cerebral cortex, the stimulus is recognized as pain and the efferent neural path is activated to provide a response to the pain. (Adapted from ASPMN, 2010)

As science has investigated and furthered the knowledge of this pain transmission theory, several other concepts have emerged:

- The central control processes and central intensity process located in the brain and limbic system help to translate the understanding of the sensation and can modulate the section of the descending pain pathways.
- When pain stimuli entering the nervous system reach critical levels, the T-cell system is activated, which creates a link between the brain and body that connects the subjective and objective experience of pain.
- By increasing the sensation of pain, peripheral nerve sensitization can be caused through continued nerve stimulation producing a state of *hyperexcitability* because of alternation in the sodium ion channels. Continued pain stimulation can be increased as inflammatory response persists.

■ *Wind-up* and *neuroplasticity* can also occur. Wind-up is a phenome-non that develops when, as the result of continued moderate to se-vere pain, the NMDA receptors are activated. These receptors serve to process the pain faster and with more intensity, creating a pain intensity that is greater than expected for the stimulus. The pain re-sponse is greatly enhanced when wind-up has occurred. *Central sen-sitization* can occur as a result of wind-up, which allows normal tissue to become extremely sensitive to pressure in areas that are not identified as painful.

Neuroplasticity is the result of moderate to severe pain that lasts for more than 24 hours and occurs in the spinal area of the nervous system. With neuroplasticity, pain fiber growth is stimulated and the pain inhibition system is damaged, resulting in more intense pain that is widespread, lessening the ability of the body to stop the pain.

Peripheral sensitization can occur as a result of neuroplasticity. This creates a condition in which nonpainful touch and pressure be-come painful (ASPMN, 2010).

As we study and begin to understand the process and theory of pain transmission, more information about the process is discovered. As science expands its understanding of the pathophysiology of pain, more information will lead to a better understanding of the trans-mission process.

The Concept of Nociception

How is pain really felt? The concept of nociception can help us determine just how pain moves through the nervous system, and it can also provide us with ideas about how we can interfere with pain facilitation and about pain inhibition. Nociception is defined as the perception of pain by sensory pain receptors called nociceptors lo-cated in the periphery. In the theory of nociception, there are four stages, or levels, of pain transmission.

1. *Transduction.* A noxious stimuli converts energy into a nerve im-pulse, which is detected by sensory receptors called nociceptors.
2. *Transmission.* The neural pain signal moves from the periphery to the spinal cord and brain.

3. *Perception.* The pain impulse is transmitted to the higher areas of the brain, where it is identified as pain.
4. *Modulation-facilitating and inhibitory input.* Input from the brain either inhibits or facilitates the sensory transmission at the level of the spinal cord. Forms the brain modulates or influences the sensory transmission at the level of the spinal cord. (Berry, Covington, Dahl, Katz, & Miaskowski, 2006; D'Arcy, 2007)

The transmission of pain is basically the passing along of a pain stimulus from the peripheral nervous system into the central nervous system, where it is translated and recognized as pain. The afferent nerve fibers are the means of moving the stimulus along the neuronal pathways.

Nociception can come from *visceral organs*, where pain is identified as "crampy" or "gnawing," or it can be *somatic*, from skin, muscles, bones, and joints, where pain is identified as "sharp." There are several different types of receptors that can trigger a pain response:

- *Mechanoreceptors*—activated by pressure
- *Thermal receptors*—activated by heat or cold
- *Chemoreceptors*—activated by chemicals, such as inflammatory substances (ASPMN, 2010)

Peripheral Pain Transmission

Pain can first be experienced by free nerve endings or nociceptors located in the periphery of the body. As a person cuts a hand or fractures an extremity, the pain stimulus is first perceived in the nerves closest to the injury. In order for a pain stimulus to be created, the sodium ions on the nerve fiber must depolarize, and this causes the pain stimulus to be initiated and passed along the neural circuitry. There are two main types of nerves that transmit pain impulses or stimuli:

- *A-delta fibers* are large nerve fibers covered in *myelin* that can transmit a nerve impulse rapidly. The pain transmitted on an A-delta fiber is easily localized and the patients may describe the pain as sharp or stabbing.
- *C fibers* are smaller and *unmyelinated*, and the pain impulse is conducted at a much slower rate. Pain that is produced by C fibers is identified by patients as achy or burning in nature (ASPMN, 2010).

Two primary substances can help facilitate the transmission of pain from the periphery. *Substance P* is a neurotransmitter secreted by the free nerve endings of C fibers whose function is to speed the transmission of the pain impulse. *Bradykinin* is a second type of neurotransmitter whose function is to participate in the inflammatory response and hyperalgesia (ASPMN, 2010). Nociception can stimulate both A-delta and C fibers for pain transmission.

Other substances that participate in the facilitation of pain include the following:

- *Histamine* is a substance released from mast cells produced in response to tissue trauma.
- *Serotonin* can be released from platelets and is produced in response to tissue trauma.
- *COX products (prostaglandin E_2 and thromboxane E_2)* act to sensitize and excite C fibers causing hyperexcitability.
- *Cytokines (interleukins and tumor necrosis factor)* can sensitize C fiber terminals and participate in the inflammatory and infection process involving mast cells.
- *Calcitonin gene-related peptide* (CGRP) is located at C fiber nerve endings and produces local cutaneous vasodilatation, plasma extravasation, and skin sensitization in collaboration with substance P production (ASPMN, 2010).

Once transduction takes place, the nerve impulse is passed through a synaptic junction from the peripheral nervous system to the central nervous system. This synaptic junction has various functions and secretes various substances. Some medications, for example *pregabalin*, act at the synaptic junction by blocking calcium channels. This in turn can reduce the amount of neuronal firing and decrease the passage of pain stimuli. The synapse is between the peripheral neuron into the central nervous system via the dorsal root ganglion.

Central Nervous System Pain Transmission

As the pain stimulus is passed from the peripheral nervous system into the central nervous system, the signal passes through the dorsal root ganglion to a synaptic junction in the substantia gelatinosa located in the dorsal horn of the spinal cord. As the stimulus pushing the pain impulse forward overcomes any opposing or inhibiting forces, the "gate" is opened, allowing the pain impulse to proceed up the spinal cord to the limbic system and brain.

The opening of the gate is controlled by a summing of all the forces involved in the conduction of the pain impulse. If the facilitating forces, neural excitability, and pain-facilitating substances, such as substance P, predominate, the pain impulse is passed on. If pain inhibiting forces predominate, the signal is blocked and the gate does not open. If by chance the pain impulse is perceived as potentially life threatening, a reflex arc across the spinal cord will fire, causing an immediate response to protect the affected area (e.g., touching a hot surface causes the body to react by removing the hand from the hot surface). This event can take place before any central processing of the neural signal.

Centrally active pain-facilitating and inhibitory substances include the following:

Facilitating

- Substance P
- Glutamate—responsible for communication between the peripheral and central nervous systems. Also plays a role in activating the NMDA receptors
- Aspartate
- Cholecystokinin
- CGRP
- Nitric oxide

Inhibitory

- Dynorphin—an endogenous opioid
- Enkephalin
- Norepinephrine
- Serotonin
- Beta-endorphin—an endogenous opioid
- Gamma-aminobutyric acid (GABA) (ASPMN, 2010)

Also performing an inhibitory role are the opioid receptors located both presynaptically and postsynaptically that are available for binding opioid substances, such as morphine, and producing analgesia. Although there are opioid receptors located at other sites in the body, those that are located inside the spinal cord have the most information available about how they function.

As the pain impulse passes through the dorsal horn, it passes across the spine to the lateral spinothalamic tracts, which then allow the pain impulse to proceed up to the thalamus and limbic system, activating the emotions and memories associated with pain, and then to the cerebral cortex, where the pain impulse or stimulus is recognized as pain. Although this process seems complicated, the body can conduct a pain impulse in only milliseconds.

Within the limbic system, two pain substances, norepinephrine and serotonin, are active. Current drug therapies, such as *tricyclic antidepressants* and *selective serotonin reuptake inhibitors* (SSRIs), are aimed at this process and use the substances to reduce the amount of serotonin available to activate neuronal firing at synaptic junctions. The synaptic junctions have such varied functions that they not only are important for producing pain but are also critical sites for reducing pain by controlling the production of pain-facilitating substances and actions.

Once the pain stimulus reaches the cerebral cortex, the afferent pathway is completed. At that time, the efferent nerve fibers are used to pass the neuronal response identified as pain back to the periphery or affected area. Descending nerve fibers from the locus ceruleus and periaqueductal gray matter are activated, and the pain stimulus is passed back down the efferent pathway, where a response to the pain stimulus, such as moving the affected area away from the pain, is produced.

Clinical Pearl	All patients with chronic pain should be assessed for depression and sleep disturbances when they are seen by their regular health care provider. Treating these conditions will help decrease the effects of pain that the patient is experiencing.

TYPES OF CHRONIC PAIN AND DIFFERENCES
BETWEEN ACUTE AND CHRONIC PAIN

A patient who has chronic pain is very different from a patient who has acute pain. *Acute pain is pain that is the result of tissue injury, such as injury* from *trauma or surgery* (American Pain Society [APS], 2008). Patients expect that when their injury heals, the pain will resolve. As the pain decreases, the patient is able to resume their normal everyday activities and level of functioning. Acute pain serves the purpose of warning the person that an injury has occurred and appropriate action is needed (e.g., treatment or moving away from the source of the pain).

Chronic pain is a different life experience. *Chronic pain is pain that lasts beyond the normal healing period of 3 to 6 months* (APS, 2008). *It is the result of injury or potential tissue damage* (APS, 2008). Chronic, persistent pain has many different sources, and the pain that the patient complains of may be in several different areas of the body. Chronic, persistent pain may exist even though there is no detectable physical source for the pain (Marcus, 2000).

The average patient with chronic pain may rate his pain level at high intensity, yet be able to function at some level. This is confusing for health care providers who expect a patient who rates his/her pain intensity at 7 out of 10 to be showing signs of severe pain, such as grimacing, moaning, or guarding the painful area. The patient with chronic pain has learned to adapt both consciously and unconsciously. Functionality is a better measure of pain relief in patients with chronic pain (ASPMN, 2010; Marcus, 2000). Physiologically, the patient with chronic pain may not have increases in blood pressure or heart rate when they are experiencing their normal daily chronic pain. Discussing the different types of chronic pain will provide insight into the causative factors for the pain.

There are several different types of chronic pain. Exhibit 1.1 identifies the two main categories, nociceptive and neuropathic pain. Figure 1.1 further classifies chronic pain into mixed and visceral pain.

Exhibit 1.1

Differences Between Nociceptive and Neuropathic Pain

Nociceptive
—Produced by peripheral mechanoreceptors, thermoreceptors, and chemoreceptors.
—Serves to warn the body that injury has occurred.
—Pain is proportionate to receptor stimulus.

Neuropathic
—Caused by damage to the peripheral or central nervous system.
—May involve an inflammatory process that perpetuates the pain stimulus.
—Nociceptive input not required for pain to occur.
—Pain is of higher intensity and disproportionate to pain stimulus.

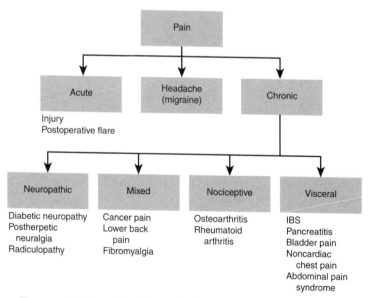

Figure 1.1 ■ Pain classification. IBS = irritable bowel syndrome.

Nociceptive Pain

Nociceptive pain is the result of tissue damage, surgery, or injury. When patients have surgery or sprain an ankle, nociceptive pain is the result. Almost everybody has experienced some type of nociceptive pain.

The stimulus for nociceptive pain is generated from various sources and specialized sites located throughout the body. Activation of *thermoreceptors* (heat), *mechanoreceptors* (tissue injury, pressure), and *chemoreceptors* (chemical irritants) can all create nociceptive pain. This means that when a patient burns a hand, has a crush injury, or has an infection, a nociceptive pain stimulus is produced. The pain stimulus is then passed along the peripheral nervous system by a voltage-gated sodium channel that allows an influx of sodium ions into the neural cell, also creating an action potential that allows the stimulus to pass to the central nervous system. Once the pain stimulus reaches the spine, if the pain stimulus is sustained, the pain signal is transmitted past the dorsal horn of the spine, through the limbic system, and into the cerebral cortex. There the stimulus is recognized as pain and translated, and an appropriate response is provided (see Figure 1.2).

Nociceptive pain is often acute and the pain will diminish as healing occurs. This type of pain serves as a warning signal to the body, which can identify the injury and protect itself. Exceptions to the short-term nature of the pain are chronic degenerative conditions such as *osteoarthritis* or *rheumatoid arthritis*, which can produce long-term pain. Outside of chronic, incurable degenerative conditions such as arthritis, it is reasonable to expect that most acute, nociceptive pain will resolve once healing takes place.

For treatment, analgesics typically are quite effective in reducing the intensity of nociceptive pain, with a 2-point reduction on the Numeric Rating Scale (NRS) or 30% reduction in intensity considered a good response. Nonopioid analgesics, such as *ibuprofen or acetaminophen*, work well for mild and moderate pain, especially that which is aching in nature or related to an inflammatory process.

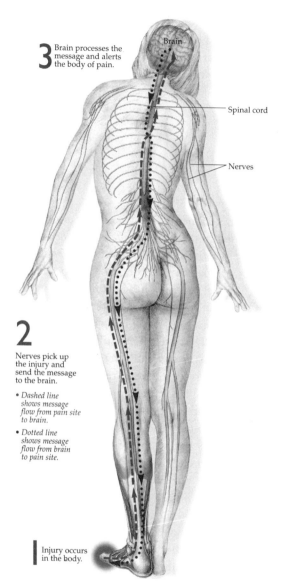

3 Brain processes the message and alerts the body of pain.

Brain

Spinal cord

Nerves

2

Nerves pick up the injury and send the message to the brain.

• *Dashed line shows message flow from pain site to brain.*

• *Dotted line shows message flow from brain to pain site.*

Injury occurs in the body.

Figure 1.2 ■ Pain stimulus process. *Source:* Used by permission of Anatomical Charts, Park Ridge, IL.

Opioids that work well for all types of pain are generally reserved for moderately severe and the most severe forms of pain.

Examples of descriptors that patients use to report nociceptive pain include the following:

- Dull
- Gnawing
- Aching
- Throbbing

Neuropathic Pain

Neuropathic pain is defined as: *"Pain initiated or caused by a primary lesion or dysfunction in the nervous system (peripheral or central) that disrupts impulse transmission and modulation of sensory input"* (Treede et al., 2008). A neuropathic pain condition can occur alone, in combination with another neuropathic condition, or with nociceptive pain. Because neuropathic pain is the result of neural damage and not tissue injury, clinical examinations, radiographic studies, and blood studies may be normal, but the patient still has pain.

Sometimes, this pain is created by a sustained inflammatory response within the nerves. Inflammation activates many irritating chemicals, such as bradykinin, substance P, hydrogen ions, prostaglandins, histamine, and tumor necrosis factor (TNF), all known to worsen pain while changing the structure and function of affected and adjacent nerves. As a result, nerve cells become more permeable to calcium and sodium channels, resulting in neuronal hyperexcitability and leading to an exaggerated response to pain stimuli (Benarroch, 2007).

Many of the abnormal processes, including inflammation, that underlie neuropathic pain operate on cyclic mechanisms that continue to spread and intensify the pain over time. Because few medications currently exist to halt the cycles that cause and worsen this type of pain, treatment is often difficult. It is very important to rule out treatable causes of the neuropathy before a final diagnosis is made of neuropathic pain.

There are two types of neuropathic pain, depending on the source of the lesion or nerve damage. *Central neuropathic pain* arises from central nervous system syndromes, such as pain that follows a stroke, multiple sclerosis, or a spinal cord injury. *Peripheral neuropathic pain* is caused by disorders affecting peripheral nerves, including postherpetic neuralgia (PHN), painful diabetic neuropathy (PDN), postthoracotomy pain, HIV-related neuropathies, and chemotherapy-induced neuropathies. Some forms of neuropathic pain have both peripheral and central nerve malfunctions generating the pain, such as complex regional pain syndrome (CRPS) and phantom limb pain.

As part of the evaluation of the patient, the painful area of the body is examined for abnormal sensations. Some patients will have diminished sensations of touch in affected areas, whereas others will have a heightened sensitivity to light touch or to hot/cold temperature changes. If stimulation that is not usually painful hurts, such as a wisp of a cotton swab or alcohol wipe, the patient is said to have *allodynia*. If there is an exaggerated response to a normally mild pain, such as a pinprick, the patient has *hyperalgesia*. These findings should verify for the clinician that the nervous system is the source of the pain.

Patients with neuropathic pain will often describe their pain as:

- Burning
- Shooting
- Painful tingling
- Painful numbness
- Strange, but clearly uncomfortable, sensations termed "dysesthesias"

SUMMARY

Although pain is a very common patient complaint, there are distinct differences between acute pain and chronic, persistent pain. Health care providers treating patients with pain should be able to recognize the differences between pain types and treat the type of pain accordingly. Acute pain may respond to typical analgesics, whereas chronic pain conditions may require a combined medication and complementary techniques plan of care. Treating acute pain effectively can help prevent the development of a chronic pain condition, such as CRPS, that can be much more difficult to treat.

Understanding how pain is produced in the body can help health care providers learn to identify the way it is being expressed physically by the patients. Patients will often describe pain as achy or sharp and knowing that different mechanisms and nerve fibers are producing this presentation can help the provider better identify the source of the pain.

The production of pain is a very sophisticated, complex process that can be difficult to understand. Learning the mechanism of acute pain production and the facilitators and inhibitory substances can help a health care provider understand why medications such as antidepressants and antiepileptic drugs can decrease pain. More information on medication mechanisms of action will be provided in the medication chapter.

Peter Allen is a 75-year-old friend of yours who lives in an assisted living facility. He is really pretty active and has been walking every night except for the last 6 weeks, when his knees began to really bother him. He fell last week while trying to get to the bathroom. He hit his elbow, fractured his wrist, and bruised his ribs and knees. When you stop in to see Peter, he tells you this is not the first time he has fallen, but it is the first time he has really injured himself.

Overall, Peter is pretty healthy with only hypertension, mild diabetes controlled with oral medications, and some osteoarthritis in both knees. Peter talks to you about the pain he is experiencing. He says,

> This is horrible pain. Nothing I take seems to help. Every time I move my arm I could just scream—it hurts that bad. They ask me to rate my pain intensity, and I always have to say 8. Sometimes I think they really don't believe me. When I'm not moving, it feels just like a toothache. I wonder why I fell? Recently my knees have been acting up, and I have this odd numbness in my feet that seems worse at night. It seems like I'm stumbling at times. The doctor gave me some pain pills, but I'm afraid to take them because I don't want to sleep all the time, and I hear about all those people getting addicted to them. I can't sleep either. There's no position that's comfortable for my arm. Is there any way I can manage this pain better?

1. What type of pain does Peter have? Does he have more than one?
2. Why is Peter's new pain so severe? Is there anything in his current condition that would give an indication of why the pain intensity is so high?
3. How have Peter's comorbidities affected his current pain complaint?
4. How has the chronic pain changed Peter's ability to function, his mood, and potentially his lifestyle?

REFERENCES

American Pain Society. (2008). *Principles of analgesic use in the treatment of acute pain and cancer pain* (6th ed.). Glenview, IL: The Society.

American Society for Pain Management Nursing. (2010). *Core curriculum for pain management nursing* (2nd ed.; B. St. Marie, Ed.). Dubuque, IA: Kendall Hunt Publishing.

Benarroch, E. E. (2007). Sodium channels and pain. *Neurology, 68*(3), 233–236.

Berry, P., Covington, E., Dahl, J., Katz, J., & Miaskowski, C. (2006). *Pain: current understanding of assessment, management, and treatments.* Reston VA: National Pharmaceutical Council, Inc. and the Joint Commission on Accreditation of Healthcare Organizations.

Bruckenthal, P., & D'Arcy, Y. (2007). Assessment and management of pain in older adults: A review of the basics. *Topics in Advanced Practice Nursing e Journal, 7*(1). Retrieved from http://www/medscape.com/viewarticle/556382

D'Arcy, Y. (2007). *Pain management: Evidence-based tools and techniques for nursing professionals.* Marblehead, MA: HCPro, Inc.

D'Arcy, Y. (2009a). Be in the know about pain management. *The Nurse Practitioner, 34*(4), 43–47.

D'Arcy, Y. (2009b). Is low back pain getting on your nerves? *The Nurse Practitioner, 34*(5), 10–17.

Fishbain, D. A., Cole, B., Lewis, J., Rosomoff, H. L., & Rosomoff, R. S. (2008). What percentage of chronic nonmalignant pain patients exposed to chronic opioid analgesic therapy develop abuse/addiction, and/or aberrant drug-related behaviors? A structured evidence-based review. *Pain Medicine, 9*(4), 444–459.

Marcus, D. A. (2000). Treatment of nonmalignant chronic pain. *American Family Physician, 61*(5), 1331–1338, 1345–1346.

Marin, R., Cyhan, T., & Miklos, W. (2006). Sleep disturbance in patients with chronic low-back pain. *American Journal of Physical Medicine and Rehabilitation, 85*(5), 430–435.

Stewart, W. F., Ricci, J. A., Chee, E., Morganstein, D., & Lipton, R. (2003). Lost productive time and cost due to common pain conditions in the US workforce. *Journal of the American Medical Association, 290*(18), 2443–2454.

Tang, N. K., & Crane, C. (2006). Suicidality in chronic pain: A review of the prevalence, risk factors, and psychological links. *Psychological Medicine, 36*(5), 575–586.

Treede, R. D., Jensen, T. S., Campbell, J. N., Cruccu, G., Dostrovsky, J. O., Griffin, J. W., . . . Sera, J. (2008). Neuropathic pain: Redefinition and a grading system for clinical and research purposes. *Neurology, 70*(18), 1630–1635.

Trescot, A. M., Helm, S., Hansen, H., Benyamin, R., Glaser S. E., Adlaka, R., . . . Manchikanti, L. (2008). *Opioids in the management of chronic noncancer pain: An update of American Society of the Interventional Pain Physicians' (ASIPP) Guidelines*. Paducah, KY: ASIPP.

ADDITIONAL RESOURCES

Ackley, J. B., Ladwig, G. B., Swan, B. A., & Tucker, S. J. (2008). *Evidence-based nursing care guidelines: Medical surgical interventions* (pp. 587–597). Philadelphia, PA: Mosby Elsevier.

American Society for Pain Management Nursing. (2002). *Core curriculum for pain management nursing*. Philadelphia, PA: Mosby Elsevier.

Dworkin, R. H., O'Connor, A. B., Backonja, M., Farrar, J. T., Finnerup, N. B., Jensen, T. S., . . . Wallace, M. S. (2007). Pharmacologic management of neuropathic pain: Evidence-based recommendations. *Pain, 132*(3), 237–251. Retrieved from http://www.guideline.gov

2

The Art and Science of Chronic Pain Assessment

THE CHALLENGE OF ASSESSING PAIN

In a recent survey of 3,000 nurses and another survey of 400 nurse practitioners, pain assessment was cited as a major source of concern and knowledge deficit (D'Arcy, 2008; 2009). Many of the nurses who responded to the survey felt that they were not getting a pain assessment that was accurate. In the nurse practitioner survey, the respondents indicated that they felt that their nurse practitioner education had not prepared them to assess or treat pain in patients with chronic pain. There were repeated requests in the comment sections of the surveys about learning to perform an accurate pain assessment and how to assess pain in patients with chronic pain and/or a history of substance abuse. Despite the years of education on pain assessment that has been provided to nurses and other health care professionals, pain assessment still remains difficult.

Pain assessment is problematic because of the following:

- It relies on patient self-report.
- Health care providers have difficulty trusting the patient's report of pain.
- The assessment process uses an objective scale to convey a subjective experience.
- The health care provider comes to the patient interaction with bias as a result of family and personal values and beliefs about pain (D'Arcy, 2007).

Pain assessment is the core component to developing and implementing care and providing adequate pain management for patients. Choosing a medication to treat pain is driven by the assessment process. Additionally, adjustments to the patient's plan of care are based on the patient's response to the intervention as determined by pain assessment and reassessment (Ackley, Ladwig, Swan, & Tucker, 2008; Berry, Covington, Dahl, Katz, & Miaskowski, 2006). If pain is not assessed well, it can result in undertreatment or nontreatment that can have significant effect on the patient.

– *For acute pain,* untreated or undertreated pain can limit mobility and result in a serious complication, such as pneumonia or deep vein thrombosis. It can also delay discharge or impair recovery and it may, in some cases, result in a difficult-to-treat chronic pain condition, such as complex regional pain syndrome (American Pain Society [APS], 2008; D'Arcy, 2007).

– *For chronic pain,* untreated or undertreated pain can limit functionality, increase the potential for disability, cause suffering, and decrease the patient's quality of life by causing anxiety, fear, depression, and uncertainty (Berry et al., 2006).

For chronic pain patients, pain assessment is more difficult because of the multifaceted nature of the pain. The patient comes to the experience not only with high pain intensity but also with depression, changes in relationships, potential impact on lifestyle related to the inability to work, and emotional needs. Conveying those varied elements of the pain experience in a single number is not reasonable. Therefore, multidimensional pain assessment scales are needed to assess all aspects of the pain experience. For chronic pain patients, functionality may be a better indicator of pain relief than a change in numeric-intensity pain ratings (Ackley et al., 2008; D'Arcy, 2007; Jensen, 2011).

Some patients do not understand the term "functionality." The term "impact on daily activity" might be better understood. Questions that can give good insight into the ability of the patient to perform the needed tasks of daily living include the following:

■ How far can you walk independently, with assistance?
■ Who does the cooking/washing/cleaning at your house?

- How many stairs can you climb before you need to stop?
- Do you go to the movies/church/visit family?
- Can you go grocery shopping?

If possible, it is always good to observe the patients while they are moving from one position to another. For example, if sitting patients are called into the health care provider's office, do they need several attempts to get into a standing position, do they use the arms of the chair to push themselves up, or do they need assistive devices to move? Does a patient limp or favor one extremity over another? All of these examples can indicate that pain is significantly limiting the patient's ability to move or function freely.

Clinical Pearl	When assessing a patient with chronic pain, always ask what the patient's worst daily pain level is and best daily pain level is. Set a pain goal that reflects a pain level that is achievable in comparison to the best and worst pain ratings provided by the patient.

Many of the original pain assessment tools were designed for research and were one dimensional, only measuring the intensity of the pain. Because of the complexity of chronic pain, multidimensional pain assessment tools are needed to assess pain. These more comprehensive tools not only include a pain intensity rating but also include questions about how effective pain medications are, the patient's mood, quality of the pain, and impact on activity (functionality). For patients who cannot self-report, such as intubated critically ill patients or demented or cognitively impaired elderly, behavioral scales have been developed to help assess pain. The following sections of the chapter will discuss specific pain assessment tools and techniques.

Assessment

Assessing pain is a subjective process; it is more an art than a science. For verbal patients, the self-report is the standard for assessing pain. To perform a standard pain assessment, the nurse asks the patient to rate pain intensity using a simple one-dimensional scale, such as the

Numeric Rating Scale (NRS). The NRS is an 11-point Likert-type scale with 11 numbers ranked from 0 (no pain) through 10 (worst possible pain) to indicate pain severity. The higher the number selected by the patient, the more severe the pain. This type of assessment is most useful for assessing pain intensity and medication efficacy.

The other basic elements of a pain assessment for verbal patients include the following:

Location—Have the patient point to the area on the body that is painful. For multiple painful areas, have the patient locate each one individually. If one area is more painful than the next, make sure the most painful area is clearly identified. If there is a radiation of pain, for example, down a leg or arm, make sure the area is clearly defined so that the correct treatment options can be determined. A body diagram can be helpful when the patient is trying to locate the pain. Using colors for pain in different parts of the body can also help determine any differences in pain intensity. Red can indicate a more severe level of pain, whereas blue can indicate pain that is less intense. Patients like to use different ways to communicate the exact location of their pain and intensity of pain they are experiencing.

Duration—Ask the patient, "When did you first feel this pain?" and "How long does the pain last?" Explore any potential sources or causes of the pain. Ask if the pain intensity varies during different times of the day and how long the periods of higher intensity pain last.

Intensity—Use the NRS to have the patient rate the intensity of the pain. If the patient has any times of the day or night when the pain intensity is more or less severe, ask if the prescribed medication reduces the intensity of the pain. If the patient is taking pain medication, determine how effective the patient feels it is in decreasing the pain intensity. Another option for determining pain intensity if the patient cannot use the NRS is the use of terms mild, moderate, or severe to see if a range for pain intensity can be determined.

Quality/Description—Have the patient describe the quality of the pain. This may be one of the most important items in the assessment process. If the patient uses words like burning, tingling, or painful numbness, it may indicate a neuropathic source for the pain. It is important to allow patients to describe the pain in their own words so it is most accurately represented.

Alleviating/Aggravating Factors—All patients have some form of home remedy for pain, and they most often will attempt to treat their pain before they seek health care. If the patient has tried some form of pain relief, ask if it helped or if it made the pain better or worse. Ask the patient if activity made the pain worse or if rest improved the pain. Ask the patient if there is any position better than another for relieving the pain.

Pain Management Goal—For most patients with chronic pain, the concept of being pain free is not a valid goal. Because of injury or continued pain from physiologic causes, the potential of removing all of the pain is very low. Work with the patient to set a goal that is reasonable and achievable. Most patients with chronic pain have a pain intensity rating that will allow them to function at their highest level. Ask the patient what pain intensity they think is acceptable and then tailor pain interventions to achieve the patient's expectations. Consistent pain reassessment will track progress toward the goal that has been set.

Function Goal—Pain is dynamic and increases with activity (Dahl & Kehlet, 2006). Ask the patient how the pain interferes with his or her activities of daily living. Assess the patient for sleep disturbances that can affect the patient's ability to function. By setting a functionality goal, progress can be tracked at each subsequent visit. (D'Arcy, 2007; 2010)

Including the patient with chronic pain in the assessment process gives the patient a feeling of validation and encourages them to work toward the pain and functional goal. Providing maximum pain relief and functionality is the goal of any pain relief treatment for a chronic pain patient (Ackley et al., 2008; American Society for Pain Management Nursing [ASPMN], 2010; D'Arcy, 2007; The Joint Commission, 2000).

The previous elements work well for patients who are able to self-report their pain. Using the hierarchy of pain assessment can help delineate the assessment process for patients who are not able to report pain.

Hierarchy of Pain Assessment

- Attempt a self-report of pain. The patient's self-report is the best way to assess for pain.
- Search for potential causes of the pain.
- Observe patient behaviors.

- Use surrogate reporting.
- Attempt an analgesic trial (Herr, Coyne, Key, Manworren, McCaffery, Merkel, et al., 2006)

In addition to the hierarchy of pain assessment, using the following basic elements in practice can help standardize the assessment process for these patients:

- Use the hierarchy of pain assessment techniques.
- Establish a procedure for pain assessment.
- Use behavioral pain assessment tools when appropriate.
- Minimize emphasis on physiologic indicators.
- Reassess and document (Herr et al., 2006; Herr, Bjoro, & Decker, 2006).

The most critical aspect of the pain assessment process for the nurse and other members of the health care team is to believe the patient's report of pain. Patients are doing the very best they can to provide you with an accurate picture of the complex pain they are experiencing. It is extremely important for the nurse to respect the patient's report of pain as presented and then, in good faith, act to help relieve the pain. If the health care provider doubts or diminishes the patient's report of pain, trust will be lost and the patient will not be open to believing that the health care provider is interested in treating and managing the pain. This lack of trust can sabotage even the best plan of care.

Most patients with chronic pain are relief seeking, not drug seeking. Approach the assessment process with a nonjudgmental attitude and a willingness to believe and invest time in helping the patient with his or her pain. The use of in-depth questions to collect all of the salient information during the assessment process will help to determine the kind of interventions that will be most helpful in providing the best possible pain relief for the patient. Using a reliable and valid pain assessment tool will provide objective criteria for pain assessment and provide a means of tracking progress toward patient goals.

Clinical Pearl	Failure to believe the patient's report of pain will ensure that the assessment process will be faulty and it will not produce positive outcomes.

PAIN ASSESSMENT TOOLS

Many of the first pain assessment tools were developed for assessing experimentally induced pain, chronic pain, or oncology pain (Jensen, 2011). The multidimensional scales were extensions of the one-dimensional scales. The multidimensional tools were developed to assess more complex pain and included measurements of mood and psychological elements. Today, there is a wide variety of valid and reliable pain assessment tools. More recently, because The Joint Commission required that all patients have their pain assessed and adequately treated, tools for assessing pain in special populations, such as the cognitively impaired, nonverbal patients, and infants, have been developed.

One-Dimensional Pain Scales

One-dimensional pain assessment tools are limited to assessing the single element of pain intensity. They are most helpful for determining if pain medication or a pain intervention is reducing the intensity of the pain. Although these tools seem very simple and the information obtained is limited, there is definitely a place for these tools in pain assessment. In a review of 164 journal articles on pain assessment, single item ratings of pain intensity were reported as valid and reliable indicators of pain intensity (Ackley et al., 2008). As an indication of efficacy, Farrar et al. (2001) determined that a 2-point or 30% reduction in pain intensity on the NRS is a clinically significant change.

Visual Analog Scale (VAS)

The Visual Analog Scale (VAS)

0| _____ |10
No Pain   Worst Possible Pain

The VAS is a 100-mm line with no pain at one end (0 mm) and worst pain possible at the other end (100 mm). The tool was designed to be used for research where a mark could easily be measured to ascertain the intensity of the pain.

To use the VAS, the nurse asks patients to mark on the line where they feel their pain intensity is best represented. If a patient marks the line at the 50-mm position, the pain would be said to be 5/10 when compared with the NRS, or moderate level pain.

The VAS is one of the most basic scales and has some limitations for clinical use.

Limitations include:
- Some older adult patients have difficulty marking on the line and place the mark above or below the 100-mm line (D'Arcy, 2003; Herr & Garand, 2001; Herr & Mobily, 1993).
- Reassessment and comparison options are limited.

The Verbal Descriptor Scale (VDS)

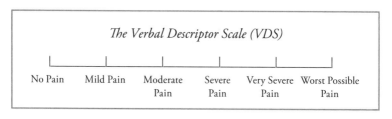

The Verbal Descriptor Scale (VDS)

No Pain　Mild Pain　Moderate Pain　Severe Pain　Very Severe Pain　Worst Possible Pain

The purpose of the verbal descriptor scale is to provide a method for patients to use word descriptors to rate their pain. The scale is anchored on one end with no pain, and the opposite end anchor indicates high-intensity pain and is labeled as worst pain possible. The scale uses words such as mild, moderate, and severe to measure pain intensity. To use the scale, the nurse asks the patient to select the word that best describes the pain they are experiencing. Clinically, some patients prefer to use a word to describe their pain rather than a number. Although the VDS is normally used for cognitively intact patients, Feldt, Ryden, and Miles (1998) found a 73% completion rate with the VDS in cognitively impaired patients.

Limitations include:
- Patient must be able to understand the meaning of the words.
- Reassessment and comparisons are difficult.

Numeric Rating Scale (NRS)

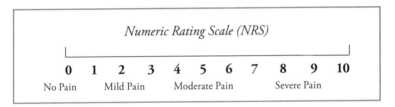

The NRS is the most commonly used one-dimensional pain scale. It is an 11-point Likert-type scale where 0 means "no pain" and 10 means "worst possible pain." To use the scale, the nurse asks the patient to rate their pain intensity between 0 and 10. The higher the number is, the more intense the pain:

- *Mild pain* is considered to be pain ratings in the 1–3 range.
- *Moderate pain* is considered to be pain ratings in the 4–6 range.
- *Severe pain* is considered to be pain ratings in the 7–10 range.

Although there is a discussion about whether a single number rating of pain is accurate, the data indicate that single item ratings can be useful. With chronic pain, the intensity rating is only one of a number of items used to assess pain. The complexity of chronic pain requires a fuller assessment than just a pain intensity rating. There is no good or bad, right or wrong number for the patient to report. It is important to believe the report of pain that the patient provides. A patient's self-report is still considered the gold standard for pain assessment.

Limitations include:
■ Only measures one aspect of pain.

Strengths include:
■ Allows for reassessment and comparison of pain scores.
■ Simple format is easy for most patients to use.

Combined Thermometer Scale

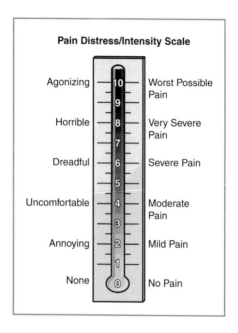

Some patients do well when they can see a graphic pain scale. The combined thermometer scale combines one-dimensional scales: the VDS and the NRS. Some patients do well with this scale and like the vertical orientation where the numbers increase from the bottom upward. The colors also highlight the increasing pain intensity as the color changes from blue to red.[1]

---

[1] The Combined Thermometer Scale appears in color on the inside front cover.

Strengths include:
- Ability to replicate pain ratings for reassessment.
- Simple, easy-to-use format.

Multidimensional Pain Scales

Multidimensional scales are used to assess patients with chronic pain with various pain conditions. The two scales that are most often used in the clinical setting are the McGill Pain Questionnaire (MPQ) and the Brief Pain Inventory (BPI). The difference between the one-dimensional and the multidimensional scales is the combination of indexes in the multidimensional scale that can utilize the following:

- Pain intensity
- Mood
- A body diagram to locate pain
- Verbal descriptors
- Medication efficacy questions

When the patient rates his or her pain using a multidimensional pain scale, there is the opportunity for the patient to more completely convey the pain experience to the health care provider. The mood scales on some multidimensional scales can help define the impact of the continued pain on the patient's personal life and relationships.

These scales are meant to measure chronic pain either for research or for clinical purposes. Another approach to assessing chronic pain that may be easier in the clinical setting is to use a set of structured questions, such as the Brief Pain Impact Questionnaire (BPIQ). This set of questions is particularly helpful for a primary interview when the patient is new to the health care provider.

Brief Pain Impact Questionnaire

The interview questions of the BPIQ capture the major elements of pain assessment for patients with chronic pain and are easy to use in the clinical setting. It is designed to be a particularly good way to organize a first assessment that can be used as a baseline. Using this format also allows the patient and health care provider to establish open communication about the pain that the patient is experiencing.

Brief Pain Impact Questionnaire

- How strong is your pain, right now, worst/average over the past week?
- How many days over the past week have you been unable to do what you would like to do because of your pain?
- Over the past week, how often has pain interfered with your ability to take care of yourself, for example, with bathing, eating, dressing, and going to the toilet?
- Over the past week, how often has pain interfered with your ability to take care of your home-related chores, such as grocery shopping, preparing meals, paying bills, and driving?
- How often do you participate in pleasurable activities, such as hobbies, socializing with friends, and travel? Over the past week how often has pain interfered with these activities?
- How often do you do some type of exercise? Over the past week, how often has pain interfered with your ability to exercise?
- Does pain interfere with your ability to think clearly?
- Does pain interfere with your appetite? Have you lost weight?
- Does pain interfere with your sleep? How often over the last week?
- Has pain interfered with your energy, mood, personality, or relationships with other people?
- Over the past week, have you taken pain medications?
- Has your use of alcohol or other drugs ever caused a problem for you or those close to you?
- How would you rate your health at the present time? (Weiner, Herr, & Rudy, 2002).

Source: Used with permission of the author.

McGill Pain Questionnaire

McGill Pain Questionnaire (MPQ)–Short Form

PATIENT'S NAME: _____   DATE: _____

	NONE	MILD	MODERATE	SEVERE
THROBBING	0) ____	1) ____	2) ____	3) ____
SHOOTING	0) ____	1) ____	2) ____	3) ____
STABBING	0) ____	1) ____	2) ____	3) ____
SHARP	0) ____	1) ____	2) ____	3) ____
CRAMPING	0) ____	1) ____	2) ____	3) ____
GNAWING	0) ____	1) ____	2) ____	3) ____
HOT/BURNING	0) ____	1) ____	2) ____	3) ____
ACHING	0) ____	1) ____	2) ____	3) ____
HEAVY	0) ____	1) ____	2) ____	3) ____
TENDER	0) ____	1) ____	2) ____	3) ____
SPLITTING	0) ____	1) ____	2) ____	3) ____
TIRING/EXHAUSTING	0) ____	1) ____	2) ____	3) ____
SICKENING	0) ____	1) ____	2) ____	3) ____
FEARFUL	0) ____	1) ____	2) ____	3) ____
PUNISHING/CRUEL	0) ____	1) ____	2) ____	3) ____

VAS   NO PAIN |——————————————————————————| WORST POSSIBLE PAIN

PPI

0 NO PAIN   ____
1 MILD   ____
2 DISCOMFORTING   ____
3 DISTRESSING   ____
4 HORRIBLE   ____
5 EXCRUCIATING   ____   © R. Melzack 1984

The short-form McGill Pain Questionnaire (SF-MPQ). Descriptors 1–11 represent the sensory dimension of pain experience and 12–15 represent the affective dimension. Each descriptor is ranked on an intensity scale of 0 = none, 1 = mild, 2 = moderate, 3 = severe. The Present Pain Intensity (PPI) of the standard long-form McGill Pain Questionnaire (LF-MPQ) and the visual analog scale (VAS) are also included to provide overall intensity scores.

Source: Reprinted with permission from R. Melzack. © R. Melzack, 1984.

The McGill Pain Questionnaire was designed to be used for pain that requires a multidimensional approach to measure pain in patients with complex conditions, such as chronic pain. Some of the areas that the pain scale has been used include the following:

- Experimentally induced pain
- Postprocedural pain
- A number of medical–surgical conditions

The tool contains a VAS, a present pain intensity (PPI) scale, and set verbal descriptors used to capture the sensory aspect of the pain experience. The tool has been widely used in various settings and found to be reliable and valid and has been translated into a number of foreign languages (McDonald & Weiskopf, 2001; Melzack, 1975, 1987).

Limitations include:
- Difficulty scoring and weighting the verbal descriptor section.
- Difficulty translating the verbal descriptor section into words that indicate syndromes.

Strengths include:
- High level of reliability and validity.

Brief Pain Inventory

Originally, the BPI was used with oncology patients to assess long-term oncology pain. With further use, it has been found to be reliable and valid for assessing pain in patients with chronic pain (Daut et al., 1983) and has been translated into various languages. It has a simple, easy-to-use format that can be used as an interview or as a self-report that is completed by the patient. The BPI includes the following:

- A pain intensity scale
- A body diagram to locate the pain
- A functional assessment
- Questions about the efficacy of pain medications

Brief Pain Inventory

STUDY ID #:_ _ _ _ _ _ _ _ _   DO NOT WRITE ABOVE THIS LINE   HOSPITAL #:_ _ _ _ _ _ _ _

Date:_ _ _ / _ _ _ _ / _ _ _ _   Time: _ _ _ _ _ _ _

Name:_ _
                  Last   First   Middle Initial

1. Throughout our lives, most of us have had pain from time to time (such as minor headaches, sprains, and toothaches). Have you had pain other than these every-day kinds of pain today?

       1.   Yes   2.   No

2. On the diagram, shade in the areas where you feel pain. Put an X on the area that hurts the most.

3. Please rate your pain by circling the one number that best describes your pain at its worst in the last 24 hours.

   0   1   2   3   4   5   6   7   8   9   10
   No   Pain as bad as
   Pain   you can imagine

4. Please rate your pain by circling the one number that best describes your pain at its least in the last 24 hours.

   0   1   2   3   4   5   6   7   8   9   10
   No   Pain as bad as
   Pain   you can imagine

5. Please rate your pain by circling the one number that best describes your pain on the average.

   0   1   2   3   4   5   6   7   8   9   10
   No   Pain as bad as
   Pain   you can imagine

6. Please rate your pain by circling the one number that tells how much pain you have right now.

   0   1   2   3   4   5   6   7   8   9   10
   No   Pain as bad as
   Pain   you can imagine

Page 1 of 2

(Continued)

STUDY ID #:_____   DO NOT WRITE ABOVE THIS LINE   HOSPITAL #:_____

Date:___/____/____   Time:_____

Name:_____ _____ _____
         Last   First   Middle Initial

7. What treatments or medications are you receiving for your pain?

8. In the last 24 hours, how much relief have pain treatments or medications provided? Please circle the one percentage that most shows how much relief you have received.

0%	10%	20%	30%	40%	50%	60%	70%	80%	90%	100%
No Relief										Complete Relief

9. Circle the one number that describes how, during the past 24 hours, pain has interfered with your:

A.   General Activity

0	1	2	3	4	5	6	7	8	9	10
Does not Interfere										Completely Interferes

B.   Mood

0	1	2	3	4	5	6	7	8	9	10
Does not Interfere										Completely Interferes

C.   Walking Ability

0	1	2	3	4	5	6	7	8	9	10
Does not Interfere										Completely Interferes

D.   Normal Work (includes both work outside the home and housework)

0	1	2	3	4	5	6	7	8	9	10
Does not Interfere										Completely Interferes

E.   Relations with other people

0	1	2	3	4	5	6	7	8	9	10
Does not Interfere										Completely Interferes

F.   Sleep

0	1	2	3	4	5	6	7	8	9	10
Does not Interfere										Completely Interferes

G.   Enjoyment of life

0	1	2	3	4	5	6	7	8	9	10
Does not Interfere										Completely Interferes

Copyright 1991 Charles S. Cleeland, PhD
Pain Research Group
All rights reserved

Page 2 of 2

Source: Used with permission of the author.

Limitations of the BPI include:
■ The patients must be able to answer questions related to their individual chronic pain conditions.

Strengths of the BPI includes:
■ It has a high level of reliability and validity.

Behavioral Pain Scales

As of 2001, The Joint Commission applied pain standards to inpatient care that have been applied to outpatient practice as well. One of the biggest focus areas in The Joint Commission standards was pain assessment for all patients, including individuals who could not self-report their pain. To facilitate the process, a group of pain assessment tools has been developed to assess pain in nonverbal patients.

The use of behavioral scales for pain assessment is one of the newest areas of focus for pain assessment, and, as such, the tools that are used are not as refined or completely developed as those that have been used for many years. The current tools are not ideal, but they are the best we have to use at this time. Some of the tools are designed to be used for specific populations, such as demented patients or critically ill, intubated patients. Although this may not seem like it applies to most patients with chronic pain, they do sometimes enter intensive care units through accident or illness, where they may need intubation and may not be able to communicate the extent of their pain.

In order to use a behavioral scale, it is important to identify those behaviors that indicate pain. The original research in this area was to develop a list of behaviors that were indicative of pain, the Checklist of Nonverbal Pain Indicators (CNPI). From the studies comparing pain in cognitively intact patients and similar pain experiences in patients who were cognitively impaired, a list of six behaviors was developed that were determined to indicate the presence of pain (Feldt, 2000; Feldt, Ryden, & Miles, 1998). The six behaviors were identified as the following:

■ Vocalizations
■ Facial grimacing
■ Bracing

- Rubbing
- Restlessness
- Vocal complaints (Feldt, 2000)

Additional behaviors that were determined to be indicative of pain were listed in the American Geriatrics Society's (AGS) guideline for treating persistent pain in older persons. These behaviors include the following:

- Verbalizations: moaning, calling out, asking for help, groaning
- Facial expressions: grimacing, frowning, wrinkled forehead, distorted expressions
- Body movements: rigid tense body posture, guarding, rocking, fidgeting, pacing, massaging the painful area
- Changes in interpersonal interactions: aggression, combative behavior, resisting care, disruptive, withdrawn
- Changes in activity patterns or routines: refusing food, appetite changes, increase in rest or sleep, increased wandering
- Mental status changes: crying, tears, increased confusion, irritability, or distress (AGS, 2002)

When attempting to assess pain in a nonverbal patients, the important elements are the following:

- Attempt a self-report.
- Search for the potential causes of pain.
- Observe patient behaviors.
- Use surrogate reporting by family or caregivers indicating pain and/or behavior/activity changes.
- Attempt an analgesic trial (Herr et al., 2006a).

Tools have been developed using behaviors to identify pain, and these assessments have been formatted in several different styles for use in varying patient populations.

Pain Assessment in Advanced Dementia (PAINAD)

Individuals with dementia are some of the most difficult patient to assess for pain. Many are nonverbal. The PAINAD is a pain assessment tool created to assess pain in patients with advanced dementia and Alzheimer's disease.

The PAINAD uses five behaviors common to patients with dementia who have pain:

- Breathing
- Negative vocalizations
- Facial expression
- Body language
- Consolability

The five behaviors are rated as follows:

- **0:** Normal, no symptoms or pain behaviors
- **1:** Occasional, slightly affected (e.g., occasional pacing, occasional moans)
- **2:** Positive behaviors (e.g., hyperventilation, body rigidity, repeated moaning, or striking out)

After determination of the extent of the behaviors, they are rated and a score is derived, providing a numeric rating for the pain. Using this tool can provide a more consistent approach to assessing pain in these patients. The tool has been found to be simple and easy to use in the clinical setting. It has also resulted in increased detection of pain.

Limitations include the following:
- Caregiver assesses for pain.
- Less comprehensive than needed for assessing pain.

There are other tools that can be used in this patient population to assess pain, but the PAINAD has been used more widely.

Payen Behavioral Pain Scale (BPS)

Critically ill, intubated patients cannot self-report pain. Many of the procedures that are performed on these patients are painful. In a large multisite study, Thunder II, pain ratings for a number of patient procedures were determined. Even so, simple tasks, such as turning a patient in bed, can result in moderate-intensity pain. When these patients have baseline chronic pain, the new pain the patient experiences is more significant and will result in higher-intensity pain.

PAINAD

	0	1	2	Score
Breathing	Normal	Occasional labored breathing Short period of hyperventilation	Noisy, labored breathing Long period of hyperventilation Cheyne-Stokes respirations	
Negative Vocalization	None	Occasional moan/groan Low-level speech/ negative or disapproving quality	Repeated troubled calling out Loud moaning or groaning Crying	
Facial Expression	Smiling/ inexpressive	Sad, frightened, frown	Facial grimacing	
Body Language	Relaxed	Tense, distressed pacing Fidgeting	Rigid, fists clenched Knees pulled up Pulling or pushing away Striking out	
Consolability	No need to console	Distracted or reassured by voice or touch	Unable to console, distract, or reassure	
			Total _____	

Source: Developed at the New England Geriatric Research Education and Clinical Center, EN Rogers Memorial Veterans Hospital, Bedford, MA.
Reference: Warden, V., Hurley, A. C., & Volicer, L. (2003). Development and psychometric evaluation of the Pain Assessment in Advanced Dementia (PAINAD) Scale. *Journal of the American Medical Directors Association, 4*, 9–15.

Assessing pain in these patients requires a tool that can detect pain behaviors, such as brow furrowing, and give an indication of pain intensity. The Payen BPS is designed specifically for critically ill, intubated patients and includes a section that is designed to assess compliance with ventilation. The three assessment categories for this scale include the following:

- Facial expression
- Upper limb movement
- Compliance with ventilation

To score each category, a 4-point scale is used that ranges from 1 (relaxed, no movement) to 4 (the highest rating, indicating grimacing, permanently retracted, and unable to control ventilation).

	Payen Behavioral Pain Scale	
Item	**Description**	**Score**
Facial Expression	Relaxed	1
	Partially tightened (e.g., brow lowering)	2
	Fully tightened (e.g., eyelid closing)	3
	Grimacing	4
Upper limbs	No movement	1
	Partially bent	2
	Fully bent with finger flexion	3
	Permanently retracted	4
Compliance with ventilation	Tolerating movement	1
	Coughing but tolerating ventilation for most of the time	2
	Fighting ventilator	3
	Unable to control ventilator	4

Source: Payen, J. F., Bru, O., Bosson, J. L., Lagrasta, A., Novel, E., Deschaux, I., . . . Jacquot, C. (2001). Assessing pain in critically ill sedated patients by using a behavioral pain scale. *Critical Care Medicine, 29*(12), 1–11. Used with permission of the author.

In the original validation study, 30 critically ill, intubated patients were divided into three groups based on sedation level: mild, moderate, or heavy. Findings from the study indicate that in each of the groups, there was a sufficient correlation with the NRS when a pain stimulus, such as a turn in bed, was performed (D'Arcy, 2006; Payen et al., 2001). The effect of the sedation was apparent, but there was still a fair correlation with the NRS, even in the group of heavily sedated patients. The tool is reliable and valid for assessing pain in this patient population. A replication study had similar results.

There are other critical care pain assessment tools, such as the Gelinas Critical-Care Pain Observation Tool (CPOT), that use behavioral observation to estimate pain intensity. Although these tools are not perfected, they do provide a means of assessing pain in patients who were once thought to be unassessable.

ASSESSING PAIN IN SPECIALTY POPULATIONS

There are some patient populations that are very difficult to assess: children, older adults, and patients with a history of substance abuse. These patients have special needs and understanding when it comes to assessing pain, and there are some tools and concepts that are helpful for these groups of patients.

Assessing Pain in Older Adults

Older patients have experienced pain before. They have any number of chronic pain conditions and comorbidities that can make selecting pain medication difficult. The older patient is reluctant to be seen as a complainer, and they may fear adding costly medications for pain to their already crowded medication regimen (D'Arcy, 2007, 2010b).

To get a good pain assessment in older patients, make sure that any assistive devices, such as glasses and hearing aids, are in place. Convey to the patients that you have an interest in their pain and would like to help relieve the pain. Educate the patients about pain assessment. Help them to understand that a good pain assessment is the best way to determine what medications and interventions could be helpful for pain relief. Include the family when it is appropriate.

Behavioral Pain Scale (Nonverbal) for Patients Unable to Provide a Self-Report of Pain

	0	1	2	
FACE	Face muscles relaxed.	Facial muscle tension, frown, grimace.	Frequent to constant frown, clenched jaw.	**Face Score:**
RESTLESS-NESS	Quiet, relaxed appear-ance, normal movement.	Occasional restless movement shifting position.	Frequent restless movement may include extremities or head.	**Restlessness Score:**
MUSCLE TONE*	Normal muscle tone, relaxed.	Increased tone, flexion of fingers and toes.	Rigid tone.	**Muscle Tone Score:**
VOCALIZA-TION**	No abnormal sounds.	Occasional moans, cries, whimpers or grunts.	Frequent or continuous moans, cries, whimpers or grunts.	**Vocalization Score:**

(Continued)

(Continued)

CONSOL- ABILITY	0	1	2	**Consolability Score:**
	Content, relaxed.	Reassured by touch or talk. Distractible.	Difficult to comfort by touch or talk.	

Behavioral Pain Assessment Scale Total (0–10)

Developed by Margaret Campbell, Detroit Receiving Hospital

*Assess muscle tone in patients with spinal cord lesion or injury at a level above the lesion or injury. Assess patients with hemiplegia on the unaffected side.

** This item cannot be measured in patients with artificial airways.

How to Use the Pain Assessment Behavioral Scale:

1. Observe behaviors and mark appropriate number for each category.
2. Total the numbers in the Pain Assessment Behavioral Score column.
3. **Zero = no evidence of pain. Mild pain = 1–3. Moderate pain = 4–5. Severe uncontrolled pain is ≥ 6.**

Considerations:

4. Use the standard pain scale whenever possible to obtain the patient's self-report of pain. Self-report is the best indicator of the presence and intensity of pain.
5. Use this scale for patients who are unable to provide a self-report of pain.
6. In addition, a "Proxy pain evaluation" from family, friends, or clinicians close to the patient may be helpful to evaluate pain based on previous knowledge of patient response.
7. When in doubt, provide an analgesic. "If there is reason to suspect pain, an analgesic trial can be diagnostic as well as therapeutic."

Source: Used with permission of the author.

Assessing Pain in Children

The two most common tools used to assess pain in children are the FACES pain scale and the Face, Legs, Activity, Cry, Consolability (FLACC) scale. Although it is not often considered, children with chronic illness can have chronic pain that can impair their ability to function normally, and their quality of life can be significantly affected. The FACES scale can be used for both acute and chronic pain, whereas the FLACC is designed to be used for acute postoperative pain.

The FACES scale uses six faces ranging from happy appearing to sad appearing with tears on the face. To use this scale, the child is asked to pick out the face that most closely resembles how their pain makes them feel. The FACES scale is a reliable and valid tool (Wong & DiVito-Thomas, 2006). The scale has also been used to assess pain intensity with non-Caucasian children and cognitively impaired adults (Wong & DiVito-Thomas, 2006).

Wong-Baker FACES Pain Rating Scale

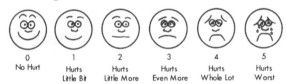

| 0 | 1 | 2 | 3 | 4 | 5 |
| No Hurt | Hurts Little Bit | Hurts Little More | Hurts Even More | Hurts Whole Lot | Hurts Worst |

Brief word instructions: Point to each face using the words to describe the pain intensity. Ask the child to choose face that best describes own pain and record the appropriate number.

Original instructions: Explain to the person that each face is for a person who feels happy because he has no pain (hurt) or sad because he has some or a lot of pain. Face 0 is very happy because he doesn't hurt at all. Face 1 hurts just a little bit. Face 2 hurts a little more. Face 3 hurts even more. Face 4 hurts a whole lot. Face 5 hurts as much as you can imagine, although you don't have to be crying to feel this bad. Ask the person to choose the face that best desribes how he is feeling.

Rating scale is recommended for persons age 3 years and older.

From Hockenberry MJ, Wilson D: *Wong's essentials of pediatric nursing*, ed. 8, St. Louis, 2009, Mosby. Used with permission. Copyright Mosby.

Assessing Pain in Patients With a Substance Abuse History

Illicit substance abuse and prescription drug abuse and misuse have been steadily increasing at an alarming rate. Patients who have a history of substance abuse are difficult to assess for pain because they often will report continued levels of high-intensity pain despite efforts to control the pain.

It can be very frustrating for a nurse to give large doses of pain medication to these patients and have the patient continue to report high-intensity pain. Some of this response is related to alterations in the patient's physiology that are created with continued use of opioid medications or illicit substances and cause the patient's body to become more sensitive to pain. This heightened sensitivity to pain is called *opioid-induced hyperalgesia*, and it can occur as soon as 1 month after opioid use/abuse begins. These patients would then report higher pain levels and require more pain medication to control their pain.

To perform a pain assessment in a patient who is actively using illicit substances or has a history of substance abuse, it is important to remember the following:

- A nonjudgmental approach is best. In order to get accurate information, these patients should feel that they can trust you with the information, and they will not be judged.
- Determine when the patient last used an illicit substance.
- Determine what the substance is and how much the patient uses every day.
- Assess for any cosubstance abuse, such as combinations of alcohol, heroin, marijuana, Cocaine, and so forth.
- Reassure the patient that you need this information to help determine what types of medication or interventions will help to control the pain.
- Reassess the patient's pain at regular intervals to determine if the pain medication has been effective in reducing pain.
- Remember that these patients may have had bad experiences with other health care providers, and try to gain trust so that they feel comfortable talking to you about their pain. (More information on treating patients with chronic pain and substance abuse will be provided later in the book.)

BARRIERS TO PAIN ASSESSMENT

Nurses still have difficulty accepting the patient's report of pain as valid and credible (Berry et al., 2006; D'Arcy, 2008, 2009). There are some barriers that make accurate pain assessment difficult for nurses.

- Bias
- Cultural influences
- Family values
- Belief systems

In order to minimize the effects of these factors on pain assessment, it is important for the nurse to recognize these influences and consciously work to derive as accurate pain assessment as possible.

Today's nurses are being held accountable for the quality of their pain management, including assessment. It is incumbent on each nurse who performs a pain assessment to attempt to get as accurate a pain assessment as possible. When pain assessment is poorly done, it can affect the patient's plan of care and adversely affect outcomes.

Focusing on pain relief as the primary end to the assessment process and treatment selection will help control fears and bias that can negatively affect patient care. Accepting and believing the patient's report of pain is essential to performing a good pain assessment. Using a recognized, reliable, and valid pain assessment tool; believing the patient; and accepting the patient's report of pain in a nonjudgmental fashion will provide the patient with the best chance for adequate pain relief.

Mrs. Livingston, age 32, is your next door neighbor. She is a single mother with two small children to support. She works a regular job at a fast food restaurant and then cleans offices at night as a second job. She does not have much time to be with her children, and she seems terribly tired all the time. She seems to be depressed about her life, and to add to her problems, she hurt her back and has been off work for 12 weeks. Her insurance is covering her medical bills, but Mrs. Livingston needs to return to work to support her family. She has difficulty in her rehabilitation related to the high level of pain she is experiencing, and she cannot always participate in her therapy as needed. The health care provider has been prescribing short-acting opioid medication to control the pain, along with a muscle relaxant. Mrs. Livingston has been advised to see a neurosurgeon to explore the opportunity for back surgery to repair the damage she did to her back. She has been told she is not a surgical candidate. At her last visit, her primary health care provider said she was becoming addicted to her pain medications and she needed to stop taking them, so he was going to taper her off the current medication.

When you speak to Mrs. Livingston about her pain, she tells you, "I know I look bad, but you have no idea of how bad I feel. I am so worried about going back to work. I need to work, but the back pain I have is so severe. At times I know I would never be able to lift the crates and stand on my feet for 8 hours a day at the restaurant, let alone clean offices. I am so depressed about all of this, and then my physician told me he would stop prescribing pain medications for me. I know they aren't all that good for you, but I really need to get back to work. I can't sleep and feel like I'm a worthless mother. I'm really caught in a bad place here. I need to work, but the pain is severe at times. Who would hire me anyway, looking and feeling the way I do. I can't sleep at night because I'm worried about my finances. What am I going to do about the pain?"

> *Questions to Consider*
>
> 1. What is the best tool to use to assess the pain Mrs. Livingston is having?
> 2. Does Mrs. Livingston seem to be evidencing any addictive or aberrant behaviors that you should worry about? Is she drug seeking or really relief seeking?
> 3. What are the biggest elements in the assessment process for Mrs. Livingston?
> 4. What could be some of the outcomes of the poorly relieved pain that Mrs. Livingston is experiencing?
> 5. Use the BPIQ to assess the pain Mrs. Livingston is having and determine what the major effect of the pain is on her life.

REFERENCES

Ackley, B., Ladwig, G., Swan, B. A., & Tucker, S. J. (2008). *Evidence-based nursing care guidelines.* St. Louis, MO: Mosby Elsevier.

American Geriatrics Society. (2002). The management of persistent pain in older persons—The American Geriatrics Society panel on persistent pain in older persons. *Journal of the American Geriatrics Society, 50*(6), 205–224.

American Pain Society. (2003). *Principles of analgesic use in the treatment of acute and cancer pain* (5th ed.). Glenview, IL: American Pain Society.

American Society for Pain Management Nursing. (2002). *Core curriculum for pain management nursing.* Philadelphia, PA: Saunders.

Berry, P. H., Covington, E., Dahl, J., Katz, J., & Miaskowski, C. (2006). *Pain: Current understanding of assessment, management, and treatments.* Reston, VA: National Pharmaceutical Council, Inc and The Joint Commission.

Dahl, J. B., & Kehlet, H. (2006). Postoperative pain and its management. In S. B. McMahon & M. Kolzenburg (Eds.), *Wall & Melzack's textbook of pain* (5th ed.). Philadelphia: Churchill Livingstone.

D'Arcy, Y. M. (2006). Pain assessment and management. In P. Iyer, B. J. Levin, & M. A. Shea, *Medical legal aspects of medical records.* Tucson, AZ: Lawyers and Judges Publishing Company, Inc.

D'Arcy, Y. M. (2007). *Pain management: Evidence-based tools and techniques for nursing professionals.* Marblehead, MA: HCPro.

D'Arcy, Y. M. (2008). Be in the know about pain management; Results of the pain management survey. *Nursing 2008*.

D'Arcy, Y. M. (2009). Be in the know about pain management: Results of the pain management survey. *Nurse Practitioner, 34*, 43–47.

D'Arcy, Y. (2010). *Pain assessment in core curriculum for pain management nursing* (2nd ed.). Dubuque, IA: Kendall Hall Publishing.

D'Arcy, Y. (2010). *How to treat pain in the elderly*. Indianapolis, IN: Sigma Theta Tau.

Daut, R. L., Cleeland, C. S., & Flannery, R. (1983). Development of the Wisconsin Brief Pain Questionnaire to assess pain in cancer or other diseases. *Pain, 17*, 197–210.

Farrar, J. T., Young, J. P., Lamoreaux, L., Werth, J. L., & Poole, R. M. (2001). Clinical importance of changes in chronic pain intensity measured on an 11 point numerical pain rating scale. *Pain, 94*, 149–158.

Feldt, K. S., Ryden, M. B., & Miles, S. (1998). Treatment of pain in cognitively impaired compared with cognitively intact older patients with hip fractures. *Journal of the American Geriatrics Society, 46*, 1079–1085.

Feldt, K. S. (2000). The checklist of Non-verbal Pain Indicators (CNPI). *Pain Management Nursing, 1*(1), 13–21.

Herr, K., Coyne, P., Key, T., Manworren, R., McCaffery, M., Merkel, S., . . . American Society for Pain Management Nursing. (2006). Pain assessment in the nonverbal patient: Position statement with clinical practice recommendations. *Pain Management Nursing, 7*(2), 44–52.

Herr, K., & Garand, L. (2001). Assessment and measurement of pain in older adults. *Clinics in Geriatric Medicine, 17*(4), 1–22.

Herr, K., Bjoro, K., & Decker, S. (2006). Tools for assessment of pain in nonverbal older adults with dementia: A state-of-the-science review. *Journal of Pain and Symptom Management, 31*(2), 170–192.

Herr, K. A., & Mobily, P. (1993). Comparison of selected pain assessment tools for use with the elderly. *Applied Nursing Research, 6*(1), 39–46.

Jensen, S. (2011). *Pain management in nursing health assessment: A best practice approach*. Philadelphia, PA: Lippincott Williams & Wilkins.

The Joint Commission. (2000). *Pain assessment and management: An organizational approach*. Oakbrook Terrace, IL: Author.

McDonald, D. D., & Weiskopf, C. S. A. (2001). Adult patients' postoperative pain descriptions and responses to the Short Form McGill Pain Questionnaire. *Clinical Nursing Research, 10*(4), 442–452.

Melzack, R. (1975). The McGill Pain Questionnaire: Major properties and scoring methods. *Pain, 1,* 277–299.

Melzack, R. (1987). The Short Form McGill Pain Questionnaire. *Pain, 30,* 191–197.

Payen, J. F., Bru O., Bosson, J. L., Lagrasta, A., Novel, E., Deschaux, I., . . . Jacquot, C. (2001). Assessing pain in critically ill sedated patients by using a behavioral pain scale. *Critical Care Medicine, 29*(12), 2258–2263.

Weiner, D. K., Herr, K., & Rudy, T. (2002). *Persistent pain in older adults: An interdisciplinary guide for treatment.* New York, NY: Springer Publishing Company.

Wong, D., & DiVito-Thomas, P. (2006). *The validity, reliability, and preference of the Wong Baker FACES Pain Rating Scale among Chinese, Japanese, and Thai children.* Retrieved from http://www.mosbysdrugconsult.com/WOW/op080.html

ADDITIONAL RESOURCES

Dochterman, J. M., & Bulechek, G. M. (Eds.). (2004). *Nursing interventions classification (NIC),* (4th ed.). St. Louis, MO: Mosby.

Gordon, D., Pellino, T., Miaskowski, C., McNeill, J. A., Paice, J., Laferriere, D., & Bookbinder, M. (2002). A 10-year review of quality improvement monitoring in pain management: Recommendations for standardized outcome measures. *Pain Management Nursing, 3*(4), 116–130.

Marin, R., Cyhan, T., & Miklos, W. (2006). Sleep disturbance in patients with chronic low back pain. *American Journal of Physical Medicine and Rehabilitation, 85*(5), 430–435.

Melzack, R., & Wall, P. (1965). Pain mechanisms: A new theory. *Science, 150*(699), 971–979.

Merkel, S., Voepel-Lewis, T., Shayevitz, J., & Malviya, S. (1997). The FLACC: A behavioral scale for scoring postoperative pain in young children. *Pediatric Nursing, 23,* 293–297.

Pasero, C., & McCaffery, M. (2004). Pain control: Comfort-function goals. *American Journal* of *Nursing, 104*(9), 77–78.

Tang, N. K., & Crane, C. (2006). Suicidality in chronic pain: A review of the prevalence, risk factors and psychological links. *Psychological Medicine, 36*(5), M575–586.

II

Pain Management Options

3

Nonopioid Analgesics

MANAGING CHRONIC PAIN USING NONOPIOID MEDICATIONS

The mainstay for treating chronic pain is medication management. Most patients expect to receive a medication prescription when they see their primary care provider with a pain complaint. However, for some conditions, such as low back pain, the current recommendations for the acute phase is acetaminophen/nonsteroidal anti-inflammatory drugs (NSAIDs) and continued activity, rather than opioids and bed rest. About 15% of the patients who have acute low back pain progress to chronic low back pain. Medication management for chronic low back pain is recommended, accompanied by a plan of care that includes medications along with other therapies, such as physical therapy and counseling (D'Arcy, 2009b). Opioids are in most cases reserved for severe level pain that is impairing functionality.

Treatment of chronic pain with medications requires a comprehensive pain assessment, history and physical examination, and medication review that includes over-the-counter medications, herbal supplements, and vitamins (Bruckenthal, 2007). Most patients with chronic pain have tried various pain medications and know which work best and which are less effective. When patients have information about medications that are effective for relieving their pain, consider this information, which is similar to what a patient with diabetes provides about daily insulin doses to a new health care provider. Just because a patient is familiar with medication names and doses, do not assume the patient is a "drug seeker."

There are genetic factors that influence the effectiveness of pain medications in a specific individual, so when patients say the only medication that works for them is morphine, it may really be a reflection of how their genetic makeup has reacted to the medications that were tried in the past. Patients should never be penalized or labeled for providing information on how specific medications have worked for them in the past.

This section will provide information about using pain medications of various types: NSAIDs, opioids, and other coanalgesics, such as antidepressants. The information will be taken from current guidelines developed by the American Pain Society, the American Geriatrics Society, the American Academy of Pain Medicine, and other national organizations (Appendix A). Included will be an order set for pain management based on the World Health Organization Analgesic Ladder and medication charts. The topics of addiction, dependency, and tolerance will be discussed in Section III. Information on integrative therapies that can be combined with medication management will be provided in chapter 6.

GENERAL GUIDELINES

All patients have the right to pain treatment, and most health care providers make honest efforts at getting the patient's pain to a tolerable level (Brennan, Carr, & Cousins, 2007). Most patients with chronic pain realize that "pain free" is not a reasonable goal to set and that a risk-benefit analysis is used to determine what type of medication management will provide the best outcome for their pain. However, chronic pain has become an extremely common patient complaint that many times requires the use of nonopioid medications, opioid analgesics, and coanalgesics. Most prescribers have very little concern when opioids are needed for short-term pain management, but when opioid therapy is required for the long-term, their concern increases, and fear of addicting the patient to the medication or fear of increased regulatory oversight can affect the prescriber's willingness to continue providing opioids to the patient with chronic pain (D'Arcy, 2009a). This can lead the prescriber to consider nonopioid medications as a first line when an opioid may be indicated. Selecting a medication that will be effective for the patient's pain complaint can be trial and error until the right medication and dose are found.

All patients who are being considered for long-term opioid therapy should be screened for risks that include opioid misuse, development of aberrant medication-taking behaviors, and addiction. The development of a comprehensive treatment plan that includes the use of various medications is extremely important to the success of pain management (Institute for Clinical Systems Improvement, 2008). If opioids are being used, an opioid agreement may be created that outlines when the medications will be refilled, the risks and benefits of the medications, the use of random urine screens, and the consequences of violating the agreement (Trescot, et al., 2008).

At the other end of the spectrum, the undertreatment of pain can produce a plethora of unwanted side effects, especially with older patients. Some of the significant consequences of undertreated pain include the following:

- Depression
- Impaired cognition
- Sleep disturbances
- Poorer clinical outcome
- Decreased functional ability
- Decreased quality of life
- Anxiety
- Decreased socialization
- Increased health care utilization and costs (American Geriatrics Society [AGS], 2002; Brennan, Carr, & Cousins, 2007; D'Arcy, 2007)

In a recent survey conducted by Stanford University, 40% of Americans in the survey reported that pain interfered with enjoyment of life and pleasurable activities and that chronic pain adversely affected their mood (Stanos, Fishbain, & Fishman, 2009). Additionally, 63% of the survey respondents indicated that they had gone to their health care provider, whereas only 31% of the patients reported that they had either complete or a great deal of pain relief. In addition, less than 50% reported a lot of control over their pain (Stanos, Fishbain, & Fishman, 2009). What this tells us about chronic pain and its management is that the problem is very big, and the ability of health care provider to control the pain is limited.

There is currently a movement among pain specialists to consider chronic pain as a disease in and of itself (Brennan, Carr, & Cousins, 2007). The effect of chronic pain on patients is so profound that it constitutes a major threat to health and wellness. Unrelieved chronic pain can affect many different physiologic systems. This includes the following:

- Reduced mobility
- Loss of strength
- Disturbed sleep
- Decreased immune function
- Increased susceptibility to disease
- Dependence on medications for pain relief
- Depression and anxiety (Brennan, Carr, & Cousins, 2007)

Because of the magnitude of the problem of chronic pain and the impact on the individual patient's well-being, health care providers need to become proficient in prescribing and dosing medications for pain of all types. The World Health Organization developed an analgesic ladder that can provide guidance to prescribers about their choices of pain medications (Exhibit 3.1). Although the ladder originally was developed for cancer pain, it has been adapted for use in many areas of pain management, including the management of chronic pain.

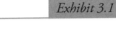

Exhibit 3.1

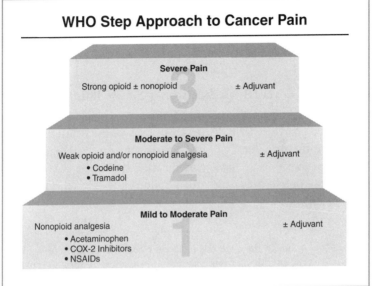

WHO Step Approach to Cancer Pain

Severe Pain

Strong opioid ± nonopioid   ± Adjuvant

Moderate to Severe Pain

Weak opioid and/or nonopioid analgesia   ± Adjuvant
• Codeine
• Tramadol

Mild to Moderate Pain

Nonopioid analgesia   ± Adjuvant
• Acetaminophen
• COX-2 Inhibitors
• NSAIDs

Level 1 Medications—Mild to Moderate Pain

Medications on the first step of the ladder are intended to manage mild to moderate pain and include acetaminophen, NSAIDs (both selective and nonselective), and adjuvant medications or coanalgesics. Adjuvant medication that can add to pain relief, although they are not primarily classed as pain medications, include antidepressants, anticonvulsants, muscle relaxants, and topical medications.

Level II Medications—Moderate to Severe Pain

On the middle step of the ladder are medications intended to manage moderate to severe pain, and include combination medications with an opioid, such as hydrocodone or oxycodone, and acetaminophen. In addition, tramadol, a mixed mu agonist and selective serotonin reuptake inhibitor, is also included in this group of medications. Adjuvant medications for this level could include the muscle relaxants, antidepressants, and so forth, of the lower level, but the acetaminophen or NSAIDs of the lower level could also be used at this point for additional pain relief.

Level III Medications—Severe Pain

Patients who are reporting severe pain require strong opioid medications for pain relief. Included in this group of medications are the opioids, morphine, fentanyl, hydromorphone, and methadone. As with the other steps, adjuvant medication should be continued to help reduce opioid needs and provide additional pain relief (adapted from D'Arcy, 2007).

> *Clinical Pearl*   Although the analgesic ladder provides some guidance in the choice of medications, the overall assessment, history, and physical examination, along with comorbidities and organ functions, need to be considered when selecting a medication for pain.

It is important to remember that the patient's report of pain is more than a number. There are many pieces of the patient puzzle that need to fit together just right to achieve effective pain management. Although the severity ratings of the analgesic ladder are a guide to choosing the correct medication because there is a group of medications in each level, the practitioner can individualize the medication selection. The efficacy of the medication is an individualized response based on the patient's report of decreased pain or increased functionality (D'Arcy, 2007).

NONOPIOID ANALGESICS FOR PAIN (ACETAMINOPHEN AND NSAIDs)

Although acetaminophen and NSAIDs are considered to be weaker medications for pain, they can provide a good baseline of relief that can help decrease the amount of opioid required to treat chronic pain. Both of these medications are seriously overlooked and underutilized as coanalgesics when higher intensity pain is reported. Multimodal analgesia, which is recommended for complex pain needs and for postoperative pain relief, may consist of any combination of medications and can include the use of acetaminophen and NSAIDs. However, there are some important considerations when adding these medications into a pain management regimen. These medications are not benign and have risk potential that should be considered when they are used with all patients. They also have maximum dose levels that create a ceiling for dose escalations.

■ *Acetaminophen (APAP, Paracetamol)*

Acetaminophen is used all over the world to treat pain. It is sold as Tylenol products, paracetamol in Europe, and is widely added to many over-the-counter pain relievers, such as Excedrin, Midol, and Tylenol products. It is available in many forms, such as in tablets, gel caps, elixirs, and as pediatric formulations. Most home medicine chests have some type of acetaminophen compound that the family uses for relief of minor aches and pains. Because it is so popular, there were 24.6 billion doses sold in 2008.

Acetaminophen is classed as a para-acetaminophen derivative (*Nursing 2010 Drug Handbook*, 2009), and it has a similar use profile to aspirin, without the potential to damage gastric mucosa (American Pain Society [APS], 2008). Pain relief efficacy of acetaminophen is superior to placebo but slightly less effective than NSAIDs (APS, 2008). The action of the medication is thought to be inhibition of prostaglandins and other pain-producing substances (*Nursing 2010 Drug Handbook*, 2009).

Advantages of acetaminophen over NSAIDs include the following:

- Fewer GI adverse effects
- Fewer GI complications

In general, acetaminophen is safe and effective when used according to the directions on over-the-counter preparation labels and any prescription-strength medication information. There are serious concerns today about acetaminophen overdoses, both intentional and unintentional. The U.S. Food and Drug Administration (FDA) has been holding hearings and is considering reducing the recommendations for daily total dose from 4,000 mg per day to a lower limit. The FDA is considering making the 500-mg strength tablets available only by prescription and limiting the number of doses in each package (Alazraki, 2009).

The concerns underlying these fears are caused by some very serious statistics about the increase in liver disease related to acetaminophen use. There is a clear connection between acetaminophen overuse and liver disease and failure. Total acetaminophen dosage should not exceed 4,000 mg per day and should include any combination medication taken by the patient that may include acetaminophen (Trescot et al., 2008). Even at this dose, there is an associated risk of hepatotoxicity (APS, 2008).

From 1998 to 2003, acetaminophen was the leading cause of acute liver failure in the United States (Alazraki, 2009). During the interim between 1990 and 1998, there were 56,000 emergency room visits, 26,000 hospitalizations, and 458 deaths reportedly connected to acetaminophen overdoses (Alazraki, 2009). Many of these overdoses were unintentional and caused by a knowledge deficit about the "hidden" acetaminophen found in combination medications. Some of the most common prescription strength combinations with acetaminophen include the following:

- Tylenol #3
- Vicodin
- Percocet
- Ultracet

Other over-the-counter medications that contain hidden acetaminophen include the following:

- Alka-Seltzer Plus
- Cough syrups, such as NightQuil/DayQuil cold and flu relief
- Over-the-counter pain relievers, such as Pamprin and Midol maximum strength menstrual formula

Care should be taken with older patients, patients with impaired liver function, and any patient who uses alcohol regularly (APS, 2008; AGS, 2009). In these cases, acetaminophen doses should not exceed 2,000 mg/day, or preferably it should not be used at all (AGS, 2009). The risk of liver failure is very real. It is imperative for all patients who are taking medications containing acetaminophen to read and understand the medication administration guidelines and recommendations. Exceeding daily recommended doses of acetaminophen can have deadly consequences.

One little known impact is the effect of acetaminophen on the anticoagulant warfarin. Careful monitoring of anticoagulation should take place when a patient is taking both acetaminophen and warfarin, because acetaminophen is an underrecognized cause of over anticoagulation when these medications are used concomitantly (APS, 2008).

■ *Aspirin (ASA)*

Aspirin is one of the oldest pain relievers known to man. It is classed as a salicylate (*Nursing 2010 Drug Handbook*, 2009). Before the beginning of modern medicine, salicylate-rich willow bark was used as one of the earliest forms of pain relief. Most Americans use aspirin for minor aches and pain, and because of its action on platelet activity, it has been promoted for early in-the-field treatment for patients who are experiencing a heart attack. It is also used for pain relief of osteoarthritis, rheumatoid arthritis, and for other inflammatory conditions but has been replaced by other newer NSAIDs (*Nursing 2010 Drug Handbook*, 2009; APS, 2008).

Aspirin is available in many different doses, but the most common dose is 500 to 1000 mg every 4 or 6 hours with a maximum dose of 4,000 g per day. It is available in buffered, sustained release, and chewable formulations.

Despite its easy availability and high usage profile, there are some serious adverse events connected with regular aspirin use. These include the following:

- Gastrointestinal (GI) distress
- GI ulceration and bleeding
- Prolonged bleeding times
- Reye syndrome
- Aspirin hypersensitivity

These reactions to aspirin are quite serious and in some cases life threatening. GI ulceration and bleeding can cause death. Aspirin is not recommended for children under the age of 12 because of the potential for Reye syndrome, which can develop when a child has a viral illness and aspirin is given for pain relief (APS, 2008). Aspirin hypersensitivity reactions can be minor or very severe. A minor reaction presents as a respiratory reaction with rhinitis, asthma, or nasal polyps. A smaller group of patients can get more serious reactions that include the following:

- Urticaria
- Wheals
- Angioneurotic edema
- Hypotension
- Shock and syncope (APS, 2008)

Although aspirin seems like a very simple analgesic, care should be taken with any aspirin use.

THE NSAID DEBATE

NSAIDs of all types are commonly used for pain that is mild to moderate in intensity. They can be used for pain that is inflammatory and as an analgesic for low-level pain or as a coanalgesic. They are available in different combinations in both prescription strength and over-the-counter preparations. They do have a maximum dose that limits dose escalation beyond the maximum dose ceiling (Exhibit 3.2).

NSAIDs have two different types of actions: selective and nonselective.

- *Selective NSAIDs* protect the prostaglandins that coat the stomach lining but do affect the other type of prostaglandins found elsewhere in the body.
- *Nonselective NSAIDs* affect all types of prostaglandins found in the stomach, kidneys, heart, and other organs of the body.

The most common use of NSAIDs is to treat pain that is caused by inflammation, such as arthritis or common musculoskeletal injuries (APS, 2008; D'Arcy, 2007).

NSAIDs have long been a standard for pain relief in older patients. Relatively cheap, they are easily accessible at most supermarkets or drug stores. They are available as over-the-counter formulations and in prescription strength as well. The most common uses are for arthritis pain, headaches, and minor sprains and strains.

Exhibit 3.2

Medication Guide for Non-Steroidal Anti-Inflammatory Drugs (NSAIDs.)
(See the end of this Medication Guide for a list of prescription NSAID medicines.)

What is the most important information I should know about medicines called Non-Steroidal Anti-Inflammatory Drugs (NSAIDs)?

NSAID medicines may increase the chance of a heart attack or stroke that can lead to death. This chance increases:
- with longer use of NSAID medicines
- in people who have heart disease

NSAID medicines should never be used right before or after a heart surgery called a "coronary artery bypass graft (CABG)."

NSAID medicines can cause ulcers and bleeding in the stomach and intestines at any time during treatment. Ulcers and bleeding:
- can happen without warning symptoms
- may cause death

The chance of a person getting an ulcer or bleeding increases with:
- taking medicines called "corticosteroids" and "anticoagulants"
- longer use
- smoking
- drinking alcohol
- older age
- having poor health

NSAID medicines should only be used:
- exactly as prescribed
- at the lowest dose possible for your treatment
- for the shortest time needed

What are Non-Steroidal Anti-Inflammatory Drugs (NSAIDs)?
NSAID medicines are used to treat pain and redness, swelling, and heat (inflammation) from medical conditions such as:
- different types of arthritis
- menstrual cramps and other types of short-term pain

Who should not take a Non-Steroidal Anti-Inflammatory Drug (NSAID)?
Do not take an NSAID medicine:
- if you had an asthma attack, hives, or other allergic reaction with aspirin or any other NSAID medicine
- for pain right before or after heart bypass surgery

Tell your healthcare provider:
- about all of your medical conditions.
- about all of the medicines you take. NSAIDs and some other medicines can interact with each other and cause serious side effects. **Keep a list of your medicines to show to your healthcare provider and pharmacist.**
- if you are pregnant. **NSAID medicines should not be used by pregnant women late in their pregnancy.**
- if you are breastfeeding. **Talk to your doctor.**

What are the possible side effects of Non-Steroidal Anti-Inflammatory Drugs (NSAIDs)?

Serious side effects include:
- heart attack
- stroke
- high blood pressure
- heart failure from body swelling (fluid retention)
- kidney problems including kidney failure
- bleeding and ulcers in the stomach and intestine
- low red blood cells (anemia)
- life-threatening skin reactions
- life-threatening allergic reactions
- liver problems including liver failure
- asthma attacks in people who have asthma

Other side effects include:
- stomach pain
- constipation
- diarrhea
- gas
- heartburn
- nausea
- vomiting
- dizziness

(continued)

(continued)

Get emergency help right away if you have any of the following symptoms:
- shortness of breath or trouble breathing
- chest pain
- weakness in one part or side of your body
- slurred speech
- swelling of the face or throat

Stop your NSAID medicine and call your healthcare provider right away if you have any of the following symptoms:
- nausea
- more tired or weaker than usual
- itching
- your skin or eyes look yellow
- stomach pain
- flu-like symptoms
- vomit blood
- there is blood in your bowel movement or it is black and sticky like tar
- skin rash or blisters with fever
- unusual weight gain
- swelling of the arms and legs, hands and feet

These are not all the side effects with NSAID medicines. Talk to your healthcare provider or pharmacist for more information about NSAID medicines.

Other information about Non-Steroidal Anti-Inflammatory Drugs (NSAIDs)
Aspirin is an NSAID medicine but it does not increase the chance of a heart attack. Aspirin can cause bleeding in the brain, stomach, and intestines. Aspirin can also cause ulcers in the stomach and intestines. Some of these NSAID medicines are sold in lower doses without a prescription (over-the-counter). Talk to your healthcare provider before using over-the-counter NSAIDs for more than 10 days.

NSAID medicines that need a prescription

Generic Name	Tradename
celecoxib	Celebrex
diclofenac	Cataflam, Voltaren, Arthrotec (combined with misoprostol)
diflunisal	Dolobid
etodolac	Lodine, Lodine XL
fenoprofen	Nalfon, Nalfon 200
flurbiprofen	Ansaid
ibuprofen	Motrin, tab-profen, Vicoprofen* (combined with hydrocodone), Combunox (combined with oxycodone)
indomethacin	Indocin, Indocin SR, Indo-Lemmon, Indomethagan
ketoprofen	Oruvail
ketorolac	Toradol
mefenamic acid	Ponstel
meloxicam	Mobic
nabumetone	Relafen
naproxen	Naprosyn, Anaprox, Anaprox DS, EC-Naprosyn, Naprelan, PREVACID NapraPAC (copackaged with lansoprazole)
oxaprozin	Daypro
piroxicam	Feldene
sulindac	Clinoril
tolmetin	Tolectin, Tolectin DS, Tolectin 600

*Vicoprofen contains the same dose of ibuprofen as over-the-counter (OTC) NSAIDs, and is usually used for less than 10 days to treat pain. The OTC NSAID label warns that long term continuous use may increase the risk of heart attack or stroke.

This Medication Guide has been approved by the U.S. Food and Drug Administration.

There are two basic classes of NSAIDs: nonselective and selective NSAIDS and COX-2 selective medications. The nonselective NSAIDs, such as ibuprofen (Motrin, Advil), naproxen (Naprosyn), and ketoprofen (Orudis), affect production of the prostaglandins that coat and protect the lining of the stomach and those that are found in other organs of the body, such as the kidneys and heart. The only COX-2 medication available at this time is Celebrex, which spares the stomach prostaglandins and does not affect platelet aggregation, so blood clotting is not affected.

Newer research from the FDA indicates that all NSAIDs, not just the COX-2 selective medications such as Celebrex, have the potential for increased cardiovascular risk, renovascular risk, stroke, and myocardial infarction (D'Arcy, 2007). GI bleeding with NSAIDs continues to be a risk; for those patients who are taking aspirin as a cardiac prophylaxis, the risk increases several fold with concomitant NSAID and aspirin use (D'Arcy, 2007).

GI Risks With NSAIDs

One of the major risks with nonselective NSAIDs is gastric ulceration. Gastric ulcers develop in about 30% of patients started on nonselective NSAIDs within a week. Most patients with these ulcers are asymptomatic and only seek medical care when the bleeding becomes obvious with tarry stools or hematemesis.

In an effort to lessen the risk of GI bleeding, some practitioners commonly use a proton pump inhibitor (PPI), such as omeprazole (Prilosec), which only provides protection for the upper GI system. Adherence of patients taking a PPI for protection is also suspect. A recent study found that by the time the patients received three prescriptions for a PPI as NSAID prophylaxis, the nonadherence rate for patients taking PPIs was 60.8%.

Because many older patients are also using an aspirin a day for cardioprotective effect, adding the incidence of ulcer formation with aspirin to the NSAID risk only increases the potential for GI bleeding.

Higher doses and older age are associated with a higher incidence of GI side effects. Additionally, chronic alcohol use with these medications increases the risk of GI bleeding and ulceration. Whether GI issues are a consideration depends largely on the individual patient's history and medical situation.

Cardiovascular Risks With NSAIDs

There are certain patient groups who are at higher risk for cardiovascular events and for whom NSAIDs are not recommended, including those patients who have had recent heart bypass surgery, patients with heart disease, and patients who have had transient ischemic attacks, or strokes. For these patients, an alternate form of analgesic is recommended.

When trying to determine which NSAID to offer a patient, consider that there are indications that naproxen interferes with the inhibitory effect of aspirin, and the same effect may be seen with concomitant use of ibuprofen, acetaminophen, and diclofenac. Overall, for patients taking aspirin as a prophylaxis, there is an increased risk of GI events, and using NSAIDs may decrease the effectiveness of the aspirin.

In general, the recommendations for using NSAIDs for pain relief indicate that the medication should be used at the lowest dose for the shortest period of time. That being the case, older patients should be aware that continuing to take NSAIDs long term for arthritis or other chronic conditions could cause serious, life-threatening effects.

New Options with NSAIDs

In an effort to minimize the adverse effects of NSAIDS newer formulations of NSAIDs have been developed to help circumvent the need for the medications to be taken orally. Some of the medications are in patch form while others are in liquid or cream form to be applied directly to the joints. These medications include

■ Diclofenac sodium (Voltaren) 1% gel. Used for localized relief of pain in joints, elbows or knees. The gel is applied four times per day and it is readily absorbed into the skin.

■ Diclofenac epolamine topical patch 1.3% (Flector). Applied directly to the site of injury this patch is used for the pain of minor strains and sprains with repeated application showing diclofenac sodium levels well below the plasma level of a single oral dose (Rusca, Mautone, Sun, Magelli, Johnson, 2008)

■ Diclofenac topical solution 1.5% (Pennsaid). A new liquid NSAID analgesic used for osteoarthritis of the knee. Uses dimethyl sulfoxide (DMSO) as a vehicle to penetrate the skin. To use the solution the patient applies 10 drops to each side of the knee with a total dose of 40 drops four times per day (See Chapter 5).

Although these medications are topical they still have the potential risks of all NSAIDs. As with all NSAIDs these topical preparations should still be used for limited time and cardiac, skin and renovascular complications are still a possibility. Patients should be educated about the potential adverse effects of these drugs and instructed to call their care provider if any unexpected effects occur.

REFERENCES

Alazraki, M. (2009). Raw risk of over the counter meds: How many Tylenols have you taken today? *Daily Finance.* Retrieved from http://www.dailyfinance.com

American Geriatrics Society. (2002). *Persistent pain in the older patient.* Retrieved from www.americangeriatrics.org

American Geriatrics Society. (2009). *Persistent pain in the older patient.* Retrieved from www.americangeriatrics.org

American Pain Society. (2008). *Principles of analgesic use in the treatment of acute pain and cancer pain.* Glenview, IL: American Pain Society.

Brennan, F., Carr, D. B., & Cousins, M. (2007). Pain management: A fundamental human right. *Anesthesia & Analgesia, 105*(10), 205–221.

Bruckenthal, P. (2007). Controlled substances: Principles of safe prescribing. *The Nurse Practitioner, 32*(5), 7–11.

D'Arcy, Y. (2007). *Pain management: Evidence based tools and techniques for nursing professionals.* Marblehead, MA: HCPro.

D'Arcy, Y. (2009a). Be in the know about pain management. *The Nurse Practitioner, 34*(4), 43–47.

D'Arcy, Y. (2009b). Is low back pain getting on your nerves? Nurse Practitioner (May) 34(5):10–7. *The Nurse Practitioner,*

Institute for Clinical Systems Improvement. (2008). *Assessment and management of chronic pain.* Bloomington, MN: Institute for Clinical Systems Improvement. Retrieved from www.guideline.gov

Nursing 2010 Drug Handbook. (2009). Philadelphia, PA: Wolters Kluwer/ Lippincott Williams & Wilkins.

Rusca, A., Mautone, G., Sun, S., Magelli, M., & Johnson F. (2008). *Comparison of plasma pharmacokinetics of FLECTOR patch (diclofenac epolamine topical patch) 1.2% and oral Voltaren (diclofenac enteric coated tablets) in healthy volunteers.* Poster presentation at the American Pain Society 27th Annual Scientific Meeting, May 8–10, 2008, Tampa, FL.

Stanos, S., Fishbain, D., & Fishman, S. (2009). Pain management with opioid analgesics: Balancing risk and benefit. *Physical Medicine & Rehabilitation, 88*(3, Suppl. 2), S69–S99.

Trescot, A. M., Helm, S., Hansen, H., Benyamin, R., Glaser, S. E., Adlaka, R., . . . Manchikanti, L. (2008). Opioids in the management of chronic non-cancer pain: An update of the American Society of Interventional Pain Physicians (ASIPP) guidelines. *Pain Physician, 11*(2S), S5–S62.

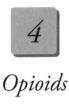

Opioids

OVERVIEW OF OPIOID MEDICATIONS

Opioids are medications that are derived from the opium poppy, *Papaver somniferum*. They have a long history of pain relief and have been used in various forms, such as elixirs, potions, and smoking substances, since the time of the Sumerians, when the poppy was depicted in art as "the plant of joy" (Fine & Portnoy, 2007). Reports from early Greek, Egyptian, and Roman societies described the fact that many of the leaders and everyday citizens used opium for pain relief. In the 16th century, the use of laudanum, an opium-derived elixir, was common for a wide variety of pain complaints. It was during this time that dependence and tolerance were noted to be occurring in laudanum users.

The term *opioid* or *opiate* denotes a class of medications that are derived from the latex sap of the *P. somniferum* or created as analogues to these natural substances. Opium has a two-sided history: one as a potent analgesic and the other as a recreational drug. For example, it was smoked for its euphoric effect in the opium dens of China and also used for pain relief. Early herbalists recognized the pain-relieving potential of opium and used it to treat many different types of pain in their patients.

During the same period, large amounts of opium were traded between the Chinese and the British. The supply was high and demand for the product was just as great, leading to wars and infighting over the use of opium to balance trade. Morphine was first isolated in 1895 in Germany, where the medication was thought to be useful as a cure for opium addiction (Fine & Portnoy, 2007). The development of the hypodermic syringe in the mid-19th century gave medical practitioners another route for delivering opioid medications, which they injected directly into the site of the pain.

By the 20th century, opioid use not only was seen as beneficial for treating pain but also had become problematic as opioid abuse increased. The United States passed the first two acts for controlling the use of these substances: The Pure Food and Drug Act (1906) and the Harrison Narcotics Act (1914). These were the first two attempts at controlling the use and prescribing of opioid substances. As late as 1970, the Federal Controlled Substances Act provided standards for monitoring, manufacturing, prescribing, and dispensing of opioids and created the five-level division of controlled substances that we use today.

In general, opioids are some of the best medications we have to control pain. They come in various formulations, and they have a good profile for adverse side effects when compared with other medication types.

Natural derivatives of the opium include morphine, codeine, and heroin. Synthetic analogues, such as fentanyl (Sublimaze) and meperidine (Demerol), were developed much later as attempts to perfect compounds for better pain relief. Several things that these compounds all have in common are the following:

- They activate by binding sites in the body called mu receptors to produce analgesia. Mu receptors are found in many places in the body, including the brain and spinal column neurons.
- Their main action is analgesia.
- Side effects, such as sedation, constipation, and nausea, are common with all members of the drug class.
- They all have the potential for addiction.

The Various Forms of Opioids

Some of the opioids are used in the natural form, such as morphine and heroin.

Other natural opium alkaloids include codeine, noscapine, papaverine, and thebaine. These alkaloids can be further reduced into more common analgesic compounds. The alkaloid thebaine is used to produce semisynthetic opioid morphine analogues, such as oxycodone (Percocet, Percodan), hydromorphone (Dilaudid), hydrocodone (Vicodin/Lortab), and etorphine (Immobilon). Other classes of morphine analogues include the 4-diphenylpiperidines: meperidine (Demerol), diphenylpropylamines, and methadone (Dolophine). Each of these compounds was developed to either increase analgesic effect or reduce the potential for addiction.

Although all of the opioid substances can be classed as pain relievers, their potency varies. Etorphine is one of the most potent of the analogue compounds, with very small amounts providing a large effect. Every member of the morphine group has one chemical similarity. There must be a piperidine ring in the chemical configuration, or a greater part of the ring must be chemically present to be classed as a morphian.

The main binding sites for opioids are the mu receptors (Holden, Jeong, & Forrest, 2005). These receptors are found in the following:

- Brain cortex
- Thalamus
- Periaqueductal gray matter
- Spinal cord substantia gelatinosa (Fine & Portnoy, 2007)

Other secondary binding sites include the kappa and delta sites. Kappa sites are found in the brain's hypothalamus, periaqueductal gray matter, and claustrum, and in the spinal cord substantia gelatinosa (Fine & Portnoy, 2007). The delta receptors are located in the pontine nucleus, amygdala, olfactory bulbs, and deep cortex of the brain (Fine & Portnoy, 2007). Recently, an opioid receptor-like site was discovered and called opioid receptor-like 1 (Figure 4.1). The activity at this site is thought to be related to central modulation

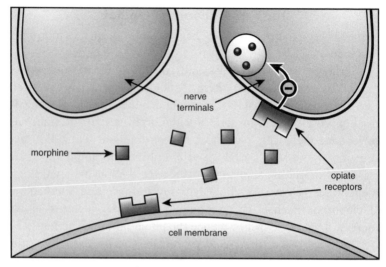

Figure 4.1 ■ Opioid receptor-like 1 site

of pain but does not appear to have an effect on respiratory depression (Fine & Portnoy, 2007).

When an opioid is introduced into a patient's body, it looks for the binding site that conforms to a specific protein pattern that will allow the opioid to bind to the receptor and create analgesia, an agonist action. At one time, the binding action for opioids was felt to be a simple lock-and-key effect: Introduce the medication; medication finds the binding site and binds, creating analgesia. Today, we know that the process is much more specific and is more sophisticated than a simple lock-and-key effect.

Once the opioid molecule approaches the cell, it looks for a way to bind. On the exterior of each cell are ligands, or cellular channel mechanisms, connecting the exterior of the cell with the interior and conveying the opioid molecule into the cell. The ligands are affiliated with the exterior receptor sites and can contain various G proteins. These G proteins couple with the opioid molecule and mediate the action of the receptor (Fine & Portnoy, 2007). "One opioid receptor can regulate several G proteins, and multiple receptors can activate a single G protein" (Fine & Portnoy, 2007, p. 11). As efforts progress to better identify the process, more than 40 variations in binding site composition have been identified (Pasternak, 2005). These differences explain some of the variations in patient response to opioid medications.

The body also has natural pain-facilitating and pain-inhibiting substances. These include the following:

- Facilitating: substance P, bradykinin, and glutamate
- Inhibiting: serotonin, opioids (natural or synthetic), norepinephrine, and gamma-aminobutyric acid

When these substances are activated or blocked, pain can be relieved or increased. These more complex mechanisms are difficult to tease out, and trying to link them to analgesia and opioid effect can be misguided. More information on pain-facilitating and pain-inhibiting substances can be found in Chapter 1.

Types of Opioid Medications

Opioid medications are very versatile in that they can be given as a stand alone medication, for example, codeine, or combined with another type of nonopioid medication, such as an NSAID (e.g., ibuprofen [Combunox] or acetaminophen [Tylenol #3 or Percocet]). Some of the medications are elixirs, such as morphine (Roxanol), and others have a suppository form, such as hydromorphone (Dilaudid). Because the morphine elixir form can be very bitter, adding a flavoring available at most pharmacies can help the patient tolerate the taste of the medication.

The duration of the oral short-acting preparations is usually listed as 4 to 6 hours, but each patient has an individual response and ability to metabolize medications. Most of the combination medications are considered short acting, and the combination of another type such as NSAIDs or acetaminophen, of medication limits the amount of medication that can be taken in a 24-hour period. Those that are combined with acetaminophen follow the recommended dose for daily acetaminophen use to 4,000 mg/day maximum (American Pain Society [APS], 2008).

Other medications, especially those on the third level of the World Health Organization analgesic ladder, have extended-release (ER) formulations. These ER formulations not only make the medication a pure opioid agonist but also extend the dosing time to 12 to 24 hours (e.g., ER morphines [MS-Contin, Avinza, Kadian] or ER oxycodone [Oxycontin]) and the new formulation of hydromorphone ER (Exalgo). These ER medications are particularly helpful for patients in whom pain is present throughout the day, such as patients with chronic pain and patients with cancer. These ER medications are not designed to be used in patients who are opioid naïve (patients who have not been taking opioid medications on a daily basis), but for those who have been taking the short-acting medications on a daily basis to relieve their pain (opioid-tolerant patients).

Some long-acting opioid medications, such as the fentanyl patch (Duragesic), have specific short-acting medication requirements before they can be used (e.g., before using Duragesic 25 mg, the patient must have been using Dilaudid 8 mgs per mouth daily, or oxycodone 30 mgs per mouth, or morphine 60 mgs per mouth for 2 weeks prior). Every patient who uses an ER opioid medication for pain should have a short-acting medication to use for breakthrough pain that occurs with increased activity or end-of-dose failure that allows pain levels to increase (APS, 2008) (Table 4.1).

No matter what type or form of opioid medication is being considered for use, the health care prescriber should be aware of the risks and benefits of each medication and weigh the options carefully. A full history and physical and risk assessment for opioid therapy should be performed.

Short-Acting Combination Medications

Short-acting pain medications come in a wide variety of types. Some are combined with acetaminophen or other nonopioid medications, and others are opioid medications, such as oxycodone, that only last for several hours at the recommended doses. For most patients with an acute injury, such as surgery, a short-acting

Table 4.1 ■ *Common Opioid Medications*

		Common Opioid Medications–Short acting	
Medication name	Generic name/ combination name	Usual starting dose–Adults	Maximum dose
codeine	Tylenol #3	30 to 60 milligrams by mouth every 4-6 hours	12 tablets in a 24 hour period Limited by acetaminophen–available as an elixir
hydrocodone	Lortab Vicodin	5 to 10 milligrams by mouth every 4-6 hours 5 to 10 milligrams by mouth every 6 hours	Limited by acetaminophen dose
oxycodone	Percocet	5 milligrams every 6 hours	Limited by acetaminophen dose
tramadol	Ultram Ultracet	25 milligrams by mouth in AM	Maximum 400 milligrams per day Limited by acetaminophen dose
tapentadol	Nucynta	50, 75, or 100 milligrams every 4-6 hours	No more than 700 milligrams on day 1 and thereafter 600 mg maximum
oxymorphone	Opana	10-20 milligrams by mouth every 4 to 6 hours	
hydromorphone	Dilaudid	2 to 4 milligrams by mouth every 4 to 6 hours	Limited only by adverse side effects such as respiratory depression, sedation, nausea

(Continued)

Table 4.1 ■ (Cont.) Common Opioid Medications

	Common Opioid Medications–Short acting		
Medication name	Generic name/ combination name	Usual starting dose–Adults	Maximum dose
morphine	Morphine immediate release-MSIR	5 to 15 milligrams by mouth every 4 hours	Limited by adverse side effects such as respiratory depression, sedation, nausea
	Roxanol	5 to 30 milligrams by mouth every 4 hours	
methadone	Dolophine	2.5 to 10 milligrams by mouth every 3 to 4 hours	Extreme care with dosing and medication initiation
			Half life ranges from 12 to 150 hours

* Acetaminophen dose should be limited to 4000 milligrams per day

Medication information taken from *Nursing 2010 Drug Handbook* and *Opioid Analgesia*, Fine & Portnoy, 2007, and APS, 2008

	Common Opioid Medications–Extended Release		

* Not intended to be crushed, chewed, or used when alcohol is being ingested

** For use with opioid tolerant patients on a schedule basis–not prn

Medication	Generic name	Usual starting dose	Maximum dose
morphine	Oramorph SR		
	Kadian	20 milligrams every 12 hours or 40 milligrams once daily	
	Avinza	20-30 milligrams by mouth daily	
	MsContin	15 or 30 milligrams every 12 hours	

oxycodone	Oxycontin	10 milligrams every 12 hours	
oxymorphone	Opana ER	5 milligrams every 12 hours	
tramadol	Ultram ER	100 milligrams once daily	300 milligrams per day
dilaudid	Exalgo	8 milligrams to 64 milligrams daily converted from current opioid doses using Exalgo conversion equivalents— give 50% of converted daily dose	
morphine sulfate with naltrexone	Embeda	Convert the patient's total daily dose of current opioid and rescue dose by 50% when initiating therapy—dose every 12 hours	

Medication information taken from *Nursing 2010 Drug Handbook* and *Opioid Analgesia*, Fine & Portnoy, 2007, APS, 2008, and PI for Exalgo, Embeda and Nucynta

In order to be considered opioid tolerant the patients should be taking at least 60 milligrams of oral morphine per day or 25 micrograms of fentanyl patch per hour, 30 milligrams of oxycodone per day

8 milligrams of oral hydromorphone per day, 25 milligrams of oral oxymorphone per day for a week or longer

Source: D'Arcy, Y., & Bruckenthal, P. (2011). *Safe opioid prescribing for nurse practitioners.* New York: Oxford University Press.

medication is appropriate, and the patient will use it intermittently throughout the period of recovery. Once the surgical pain resolves, the patient does not need to take the opioid medication any longer and stops medication use. Patients with chronic pain require a more complex medication regimen to control their pain effectively.

Most short-acting medications are oral, as either pills or elixirs. For surgical pain, a short-acting medication may be needed in the immediate postoperative period, and these are given as intermittent intravenous (IV) doses or through epidural or patient-controlled analgesia. One route of administration that is no longer recommended is the intramuscular (IM) route. Because the administration of medication via the IM route allows for irregular absorption and tissue sclerosis, most national guidelines and pain specialists have eliminated the IM route from their recommendations (APS, 2008).

For patients with chronic pain, the pain will continue with no end point, and so medication use will continue. For these patients, a careful assessment of pain patterns and intensities throughout the day will help determine when and how the opioid medication will be prescribed. For some patients with chronic pain, sitting can be very painful, whereas others cannot tolerate standing or lying in bed. For these patients, pain medication should be chosen to have the biggest effect on these particularly painful times. If the pain is only episodic or present at certain times of day, a short-acting medication may provide all the pain relief that is needed. However, most patients with chronic pain have pain that is continuous, so adding an ER medication is common.

Most short-acting opioid medications are designed for moderate to severe pain intensities. Onset of action is usually 10 to 60 minutes, with a short duration of action of 2 to 4 hours (Katz, McCarberg, & Reisner, 2007). Overall advantages to short-acting medications include a synergistic effect with the combination medications such as acetaminophen and an opioid, that can improve pain relief and provide a better outcome.

MEDICATIONS

Short-Acting Combination Medications: Intermittent Pain and Breakthrough Pain

■ *Codeine-Containing Medications: Codeine and Tylenol #3 (Codeine 30 mg Combined With Acetaminophen 325 mg)*

Used to treat mild to moderate pain, codeine[1] is noted to have a number needed to treat of 11. That means the first effective analgesic effect would be seen in the 12th patient who was given the medication for pain relief. About 10% of the people lack the enzyme needed to activate codeine (APS, 2008). Codeine has a high profile for side effects, such as constipation and gastrointestinal (GI) disturbances, including nausea and vomiting (APS, 2008). It is often used as a component in cough syrups as a cough suppressant (*Nursing 2010 Drug Handbook*, 2009), and the medication can be given in an elixir form, which is convenient for patients who have difficulty swallowing or for use with enteral feeding tubes.

■ *Hydrocodone-Containing Medications: Vicodin, Lortab, Norco, and Lortab Elixir*

Hydrocodone-containing medications are designed to be used for moderate pain. They usually contain 5 to 10 mg of hydrocodone with 325 mg or 500 mg of acetaminophen. Many patients tolerate the medication very well for intermittent pain or for breakthrough pain. It has an Elixir form that is very effective and can be used in patients who have difficulty swallowing pills or who have enteral feeding tubes. Norco has a higher dose of hydrocodone per tablet.

■ *Oxycodone-Containing Medications: Oxycodone, Percocet, Roxicet, Percodan, and Oxyfast*

Medications with oxycodone are designed to treat moderate-level pain. They are commonly used for postoperative pain in the acute care setting and for patients with chronic pain. Percocet is a combination medication with 5 mg of oxycodone and 325 mg of acetaminophen.

---

[1] Codeine should be used with caution in breastfeeding women who may inadvertently give their infants a morphine overdose if they are ultrarapid codeine metabolizers (*Nursing 2010 Drug Handbook*, 2009).

Percodan is combined with aspirin in place of acetaminophen in Percocet. If the patient requires a higher dose of medication for pain control,
administering an oxycodone 5 mg tablet with a combined form, such as
Roxicet, will provide additional pain relief but still maintain the acetaminophen dose at 325 mg. To help patients tolerate the medication
without nausea, giving the medication with milk or after meals is recommended (*Nursing 2010 Drug Handbook*, 2009).

■ *Oxymorphone-Containing Medications: Opana*

Opana is a medication designed to treat moderate to severe pain.
The medication has a more extended half-life than other medications of the same class, resulting in a decreased need for breakthrough medications. The medication should be taken 1 hour before
or 2 hours after a meal (*Nursing 2010 Drug Handbook*, 2009). It is also
available in an injectable form for use during labor (*Nursing 2010
Drug Handbook*, 2009).

■ *Tramadol: Ultram and Ultracet*

Tramadol is a rather unique combination medication. It is a combination of a mu agonist, an opioid-like medication, and a selective serotonin reuptake inhibitor–type medication. It is designed for use with
moderate pain. Doses should be reduced for older patients and in patients with increased creatinine levels or cirrhosis. Tramadol may increase the risk of seizures and serotonin syndrome (*Nursing 2010 Drug
Handbook*, 2009). Patients should be instructed to taper off tramadol
gradually when discontinuing the medication. It should not be stopped
suddenly (*Nursing 2010 Drug Handbook*, 2009). A new medication, tap-
entadol (Nucynta), with similar action has just been released.

■ *Hydromorphone: Dilaudid*

Dilaudid is an extremely potent analgesic and it is designed for use with
severe level pain. In the oral form, it comes in 2 mg and 4 mg tablets. In
the IV form, 0.2 mg of Dilaudid is equal to 1 mg of IV morphine. Dilaudid
is a medication that is commonly used after the usual medications for
pain (e.g., Vicodin and Percocet) are trialed unsuccessfully. Because of
the strength of this medication, it is possible to give small amounts, get
good pain relief, and potentially have fewer side effects.

■ *Morphine: Immediate-Release Morphine (MSIR) and Roxanol (Elixir)*

Morphine is the gold standard for pain relief. It is the standard for equianalgesic conversions and has a long history of use in many different forms for pain control. It is available as pills, elixir, IV, and suppository. It is indicated for severe level pain. The biggest drawback to morphine is the side effect profile; constipation, nausea and vomiting, delirium, and hallucinations are some of the most commonly reported adverse effects.

■ *Fentanyl Transmucosal (Sublimaze): Actiq, Fentora, and Onsolis*

There is no oral pill formulation possible for fentanyl. The route of administration is either transdermal or buccal. When used buccally for breakthrough pain in opioid-tolerant patients, the transmucosal medications can be rubbed across the buccal membrane and absorbed directly into the cardiac circulation. The fast absorption makes this medication a risk for oversedation, so the indication is only for breakthrough pain in opioid-tolerant cancer patients or patients with chronic pain who take opioid medications on a daily basis.

If the entire dose of an Actiq Oralet is not used, it should be placed in a childproof container until the remainder is needed. This medication is not meant to be used for acute or postoperative pain (*Nursing 2010 Drug Handbook*, 2009). It is not meant to be used in opioids-naïve patients because serious oversedation can occur (Fine & Portnoy, 2007).

Extended-Release Medications: Pain Relief for Consistent Pain and Around-the-Clock Pain Relief

For patients with chronic pain, ER medication can give a consistent blood level of medication that can provide a steady comfort level. This may increase functionality and improve quality of life, enhance sleep, and let the patient participate in meaningful daily activities. ER medications have a slower onset of action of about 30–90 minutes, with a relatively long duration of action up to 72 hours (Katz, McCarberg, & Reisner, 2007).

When a patient has pain that lasts throughout the day and the patient is taking short-acting medications and has reached the maximum dose limitations of the nonopioid component in the medication, the prescriber should consider switching the patient to an ER or long-acting medication. Some of the short-acting medications have an ER formulation (e.g., Vicodin ER, Opana ER, Ultram ER, Oxycontin, Kadian, Avinza, and MS-Contin, Embedda, Exalgo). Most are pure mu agonist medications, such as morphine, with an ER action that allows the medication, to dissolve slowly in the GI tract. Some ER medications are encapsulated into beads that allow gastric secretions to enter the bead and force the medication out. Other ER formulations have a coating around an ER plasticized compound that keeps the medication from dissolving too quickly Embedda is a new morphine formulation that has a core of naltrexone, a mu antagonist or reversal agent, in each pellet in the capsule. The naltrexone is released if the pellet is crushed or chewed. If the tablet is taken correctly the naltrexone passes through the GI system and is excreted unused. By adding the naltrexone core to the medication pellets, diversion and tampering is discouraged. When ER medication is being started in a patient, the patient should be instructed on the important aspects of the medications. Important information includes the following:

- ER medications of all types should never be broken, chewed, or degraded in any way to enhance the absorption of the medications. To do so risks all the medication being given at one time, and there is then a high risk of potentially fatal oversedation.
- Most ER medications should not be taken with alcohol. To do so degrades the ER mechanism and allows for a faster absorption of the medication, which can cause potentially fatal oversedation.
- ER medications are not meant to be injected.
- ER medication should not be crushed and inserted into enteral feeding tubes.
- ER medications are not meant to be used on an as-needed basis but rather in scheduled daily doses (APS, 2008).
- If the patient experiences end-of-dose failure several hours before the next dose of medication is due, the interval should be shortened or the dose should be increased (APS, 2008).

When converting a patient from short-acting medications, the rule of thumb is the following:

- If the medication is the same drug, Percocet to Oxycontin for example, equivalent doses of the medication can be prescribed.

■ If the medication is a different drug, Percocet to MS-Contin for example, the daily dose should be calculated using the equianalgesic conversion table (see Appendix B) and reduced usually by 30%. To ensure adequate pain relief is maintained, additional doses of breakthrough medication should be prescribed at about 5% to 15% of the total daily dose to be taken every 2 hours as needed (APS, 2008).

■ *Methadone: Dolophine and Methadose*

Methadone is considered to be a long-acting medication because it has an extended half-life of 15 to 60 hours (APS, 2008). Pain relief, however, for the oral form is less extended at 4 to 6 hours (*Nursing 2010 Drug Handbook*, 2009). Therein lies the danger. If the half-life is very long and the pain relief is shorter, dosing must be done very carefully to avoid oversedating the patient, which may become apparent only a day or two after the doses are given. Dose escalation should be done no more often than every 3–7 days.

Methadone can be prescribed legally by general practitioners in primary care for pain relief. It is also used in methadone maintenance programs to control addiction in heroin addicts. Prescribing methadone for these patients requires a special licensure. The addiction program has no connection to prescribing methadone for pain management. However, because there is such a risk with this medication, the current recommendation of the APS is that only pain management practitioners or those skilled and knowledgeable about the medication prescribe the drug (D'Arcy, 2009a).

An additional risk factor for this medication is the potential for QT interval prolongation and, with higher doses, for torsades de pointes (APS, 2008). Primary care providers are advised to obtain a baseline electrocardiogram (ECG) for patients who are on daily methadone and continue to obtain regular ECGs as the doses escalate above 200 mg/day (APS, 2008).

■ *Fentanyl Patches: Duragesic*

Fentanyl patches can provide a high level of pain relief and are used for various chronic pain conditions. These patches are the only transdermal opioid application that is available for use. The Duragesic patch is a delivery system that contains a specified dose of fentanyl in a gel formulation. It is designed for use with opioid-tolerant patients and should never be used for acute pain or with opioid-naïve patients.

The patch is applied to clean intact skin and delivers the specified amount of medication for 72 hours (e.g., 25 mcg/h). The medication effect begins as the medication depot develops in the subcutaneous fat, and it can take from 12 to 18 hours for pain relief to begin. It can also take up to 48 hours for steady-state blood levels to develop, so when the patch is being started, the patient will need additional break-through pain medication to control pain (D'Arcy, 2009a).

There are some safety concerns with Duragesic patch use. More than 100 patient deaths have been linked to fentanyl patch use and misuse. When a patch is prescribed for pain relief, the education of the patients should include the following:

- Do not cut the patch. To do so will cause a dose-dumping effect in which all the medication is released at one time, resulting in an overdose.
- Do not apply heat over the patch. To do so may cause accelerated medication delivery, also resulting in overdose.
- Dispose of the patch in a closed container, flush it down a toilet, or seal it in a bag with kitty litter or used coffee grounds. Safe disposal is necessary to avoid diversion and minimize contamination.
- Do not place the patch in a regular wastebasket when discarding it. There is about 16% of the dose remaining in the patch after use, and a small animal or child could remove the patch and chew or place it on him- or herself, resulting in overdose.
- To receive a 25 mcg fentanyl patch, the patient should be taking one of the following: 30 mg of oxycodone per day for 2 weeks, 8 mg of hydromorphone per day for 2 weeks, or 60 mg of oral morphine per day for 2 weeks.

Medications That Are No Longer Recommended

There are two pain medications that are no longer recommended for use because of toxic metabolites, high acetaminophen doses, or high profile for side effects.

■ *Propoxyphene: Darvocet*

Darvocet is a medication that has fallen out of favor and is being considered for withdrawal by the U.S. Food and Drug Administration because of the high levels of acetaminophen and a toxic metabolite called norpropoxyphene. The medication contains 650 mg of acetaminophen and 50 or 100 mg of propoxyphene in each tablet. It is designed to treat mild level pain, but its analgesic action is created primarily by the high dose of acetaminophen in each tablet. It is very easy to reach daily maximum doses of acetaminophen with just a few tablets of Darvocet. Additionally, there is a toxic metabolite called norpropoxyphene that builds up with use. The effect of the norpropoxyphene is to cause seizures (APS, 2008). For this reason, it is not used very often by pain specialists for pain control, and it is not recommended for patients with renal impairment or older adults (APS, 2008).

■ *Meperidine: Demerol*

Meperidine (Demerol) has also fallen out of favor. It is no longer considered a first-line pain medication (APS, 2008). Meperidine has a toxic metabolite called normeperidine that accumulates with repetitive dosing (APS, 2008). This metabolite can cause tremors and seizures. Other drawbacks include the need to use high doses to achieve an analgesic effect that is accompanied by sedation and nausea. If Demerol is going to be used, there are certain recommendations that include the following:

- Demerol should never be used in children and infants.
- It should never be used in patients with renal impairment (e.g., patients with sickle-cell disease or older patients).
- Hyperpyrexic syndrome with delirium can occur if Demerol is used in patients who are taking monoamine oxidase inhibitors, which can be potentially fatal.
- If used, it should never be for more than 1 to 2 days at doses not to exceed 600 mg/24 h (APS, 2008).

Mixed Agonists/Antagonist Medications

There is a group of medications that have both an agonist and antagonist action at the various binding sites throughout the body. These medications are called *mixed agonist/antagonist medications.* These medications include the following:

- Nubain
- Talwin
- Buprenex

These medications act further down on the spinal cord at the kappa receptor sites, so the potential for respiratory depression is felt to be less. Because these medications have both agonist and antagonist action, they have the potential for reversing the opioid effect of pure opioid agonists, such as morphine. If a patient is taking morphine, giving a mixed agonist/antagonist medication will reverse the effect of the morphine and pain relief is lessened. This group of medications also has a high profile for adverse side effects, such as confusion and hallucinations, and has dose ceilings that limit dose escalations (APS, 2008).

Selecting an Opioid

Selecting an opioid for an individual patient can involve a trial-and-error process. Each individual has an unknown genetic preference for one or more types of opioids. It is a process of determining which opioid works best for the patient.

Many patients with chronic pain have tried opioids before. They may know which ones work best and which ones do not work at all. If the patient can provide information on the efficacy of pain medications, it should not be considered as drug seeking or potential addiction. If the patient has used a medication successfully, starting with one that was effective will, in many cases, provide the best outcome.

Conversely, if the patient says that he or she has tried a medication but that it did not work, get more information about when, for what indication, and what doses were tried. In many cases, patients with chronic pain have been underdosed with medications, and they then feel the medications are "not working" or are ineffective. If the correct dose of medication had been provided, the medication could have provided good pain relief. It is always wise to revisit the use of a medication that has been underdosed by using appropriate doses for treating pain unless there are side effects that would contraindicate the use of the drug (Figure 4.2).

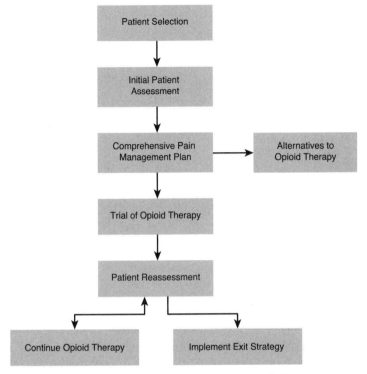

Figure 4.2 ■ Algorithm for opioid treatment of chronic pain

Opioids in the Older Patient

Older patients have a higher occurrence of painful conditions, such as osteoarthritis and other comorbidities. Choosing a medication to manage pain in these patients can be a complex challenge. The myth that older patients do not tolerate pain medications is just that, a myth. Older patients can use even opioid medication with good effect if careful dosing and titration take place.

The American Geriatrics Society (AGS) has released a new set of pain management guidelines for persistent pain in older patients (2009). These new guidelines indicate that opioids are an option for the older patient when moderate to severe pain is present.

For older patients, pain is experienced in much the same way as younger patients, but aging can change the way the nervous system perceives the pain and transmission may be altered. Aging can also change the way the older patient's body processes pain medications and can increase the potential for adverse effects. Some of the reasons an older patient may experience adverse effects include the following:

- Muscle-to-fat ratios change as patients age, causing the body fat composition to be altered.
- Poor nutrition can decrease protein stores, which in turn can decrease the binding ability of some medications.
- Because of the changes in the protein-binding mechanisms, drugs may need to compete for binding sites, making one or more of the patient's medications ineffective.
- Aging affects the physiologic functions of metabolism, absorption, medication clearance, including a slowed GI motility, decreased cardiac output, and decreased glomerular filtration rate.
- Baseline changes in sensory and cognitive perception, such as sedation or confusion related to opioid use, can be an increased risk for some patients.
- Drug excretion and elimination are reduced by 10% for each decade after 40 years of age because of decreased renal function (Taken from-Bruckenthal & D'Arcy, 2007; D'Arcy, 2009b).

The old adage of starting low and going slow still applies to opioid therapy in older adults. Older patients are not all the same, and bodies age in different ways. Using conservative doses and monitoring the patient carefully for side effects can help ensure that opioids are being used to provide the highest possible pain relief but that the medication is also being used safely.

Tips for Starting Analgesic Medication in the Older Patient

Because the older patient has pain needs that require more monitoring of dosing and adverse effects, starting new medications can be somewhat complicated. Recommendations for pain medications for the older adult include the following:

- Decrease acetaminophen dose if the patient has a history of alcohol use/abuse or liver or renal impairment. The maximum daily dose should be decreased by 50% to 75% from 4 g/day or not used at all (AGS, 2009).
- Reduce beginning opioid doses by 25% to 50% to decrease the potential for oversedation.
- Scheduling medication may provide better pain relief and reduce the likelihood of needing increased doses for uncontrolled pain.
- Monitor older adults being started on opioid therapy daily if not more frequently because organ impairment may decrease the elimination of the medication.
- Avoid the use of the following medications because of unwanted side effects and/or toxic metabolites: meperidine, propoxyphene, pentazocine, indomethacin, and amitriptyline. (D'Arcy, 2010)

Managing Side Effects of Opioid Treatment

All opioids have the potential for side effects. There is no magic opioid or pain medication that does not have the potential for constipation, sedation, or pruritus. Opioids can be used in the presence of side effects, but treatment options to control the unwanted effects or dose reductions to minimize the side effects should be used. One important concept to remember here is that adding a medication that is sedating, such as promethazine, can potentiate sedation from an opioid. Before deciding that an opioid is too sedating, look at all sedating medications that are being used concomitantly and try to minimize the use of additional sedating agents.

Constipation

Constipation is a common side effect of opioid use. It is the one effect to which the patient will not become tolerant. Every patient who is prescribed an opioid should have a laxative of some type. Stool softeners are also used to ease bowel movement. Stimulant laxatives are used to counteract the constipation. Combination stool softener/ laxatives are available over the counter in most drugstores. Recommended types of laxatives include the following:

- Senna or Senna with stool softener—increases bowel motility
- bisacodyl—increases bowel motility
- Lactulose—osmotic laxative
- Sorbitol—easily found in Sorbee candies; osmotic laxative
- methylnaltrexone (Relistor)—approved for opioid-induced constipation for patients with advanced illness or palliative care; subcutaneous injectable (APS, 2008)

Sedation

Patients may become sedated when opioids are first started, but they become tolerant to the effect within a period of 2 weeks or less. If sedation persists or sedation reaches high levels, dose adjustments should be made so that serious oversedation does not occur. Sedation occurs most commonly at the beginning of opioid therapy. Patients should be monitored for sedating effects of the opioid and additive sedating effects from medications that are sedating, such as antiemetics, sedatives, antihistamines, muscle relaxants, sleeping medications, benzodiazepines, and so forth.

To counteract sedation, stimulants such as caffeine, dextroamphetamine, methylphenidate, or modafinil can be used. The medications listed previously are most commonly used for patients with chronic cancer pain. Most patients adjust to the sedating effects of opioids within a few weeks at the longest, but the use of caffeine can be recommended for almost any patient.

Pruritus (Itching)

Some patients who started on opioids or are taking high doses of opioids may develop pruritus, commonly known as itching. It was once thought to be caused by a histamine release but the true source of the condition is undetermined and it is not an indication of a true allergy. The most common way to counteract the itching is to use an antihistamine, such as diphenhydramine (Benadryl). If the itching persists, changing to another opioid may reduce or eliminate this effect.

Delirium/Confusion

Many patients, especially older patients, become confused when they are moved from their usual living situation and put into a new situation or have surgery and start opioids. Delirium can be caused by opioids, and it is a temporary state. If the patient becomes delirious, changing the opioid, reducing the dose, or stopping the opioid may provide the needed intervention. Some opioids, such as morphine, have a higher profile for confusion. Changing to another medication, such as low-dose Dilaudid, may provide adequate pain relief and lessen the potential for confusion.

Nausea and Vomiting

Opioids have a high profile for nausea and vomiting. For most opioids, taking the medication with a small amount of food or milk will help to reduce the effect. If the nausea and vomiting do not resolve, using an antiemetic regularly until the effect abates is the best option. Because all antiemetics are sedating, there will be an addictive sedating effect when the medications are combined. Recommended antiemetics include the following:

- ondansetron
- Phenergan[2]
- Reglan
- For motion-induced nausea: meclizine or cyclizine
- For severe cases: scopolamine patches (APS, 2008)

---

[2] Phenergan should be used with caution with IV administration. This medication can cause tissue necrosis.

Peter Simmons, age 48, is an over-the-road truck driver. He was involved in a four-wheel roll over accident more than 8 months ago while he was on vacation in Montana. He has had two surgeries to repair the back injuries he sustained in the accident, but now he is left with residual low back pain that radiates down his left leg. He rates his pain at 8/10. He is currently taking 6 Percocet per day, as well as a muscle relaxant. He finds it very difficult to participate in physical therapy, and he has not been able to work since the accident. He is unable to sleep, and he has lost 20 lb since the accident. His primary care physician sends Peter to you, a pain specialist, to see if there is anything that can be done about improving his pain management.

When you interview Peter, he tells you, "I wish I'd never gotten on that four-wheeler. I had no idea it would roll over that way. Now all I have is pain, and I can't do anything anymore. I absolutely cannot stand or sit down. The pain becomes unbearable. I have to lie on the couch all day and most of the night to get any relief. My wife can't understand why no one can fix the pain. She and I argue a lot now. I take my pain medications, but they don't seem to help. My left leg has a burning pain that just streaks down my leg when I try to put pressure on it. I'll never be able to drive truck again. Now, how am I going to support my family?"

RECOMMENDATIONS

- Begin an ER pain medication, such as Oxycontin or MS-Contin.
- Add a neuropathic pain medication, such as Lyrica, Neurontin, or Cymbalta.
- Continue the Percocet for breakthrough pain.
- Continue the muscle relaxant for muscle spasms.
- Send Peter for a modified physical therapy regimen or a multidisciplinary pain rehabilitation program.

Questions to Consider

1. Is using an extended release pain medication indicated for Peter? If yes, why?
2. What role is the depression and anxiety Peter feels about the loss of his job playing in the scenario? What about his relationship with his wife? Is an antidepressant indicated?
3. Is Cymbalta a good choice for Peter's leg pain and depression?
4. Will Peter continue to need opioid medications or is there a possibility that he could be converted to nonopioid medications?
5. How would you decide if Oxycontin or MS-Contin is the best choice for Peter?

REFERENCES

American Geriatrics Society. (2009). *Persistent pain in the older patient.* Retrieved from www.americangeriatrics.org

American Pain Society. (2008). *Principles of analgesic use in the treatment of acute pain and cancer pain.* Glenview, IL: Author.

D'Arcy, Y. (2007). *Pain management: Evidence-based tools and techniques for nursing professionals.* Marblehead, MA: HCPro.

D'Arcy, Y. (2009a). Avoid the dangers of opioid therapy. *American Nurse Today, 4*(5), 16–22.

D'Arcy, Y. (2009b). *Pain in the older adult.* Indianapolis, IN: Sigma Theta Tau.

Fine, P. G., & Portnoy, R. (2007). *A clinical guide to opioid analgesia.* New York, NY: Vendome Group.

Holden, J., Jeong, Y., & Forrest, J. (2005). The endogenous opioid system and clinical pain management. *AACN Clinical Issues, 16*(3), 291–301.

Katz, N., McCarberg, B., & Reisner, L. (2007). *Managing chronic pain with opioids in primary care.* Newton, MA: Inflexxion.

Nursing 2010 Drug Handbook. (2009). Philadelphia, PA: Lippincott Williams & Wilkins.

Pasternak, G. W. (2005). Molecular biology of opioid analgesia. *Journal of Pain and Symptom Management, 29*(Suppl. 5), S2–S9.

ADDITIONAL RESOURCES

Chou, R., Fanciullo, G., Fine, P., Adler, J., Ballantyne, J., Davies, P., . . . American Pain Society–American Academy of Pain Medicine Opioids Guidelines Panel. (2009). Clinical guidelines for the use of chronic opioid therapy in chronic noncancer pain. *The Journal of Pain, 10*(2), 113–130.

Fine, P. G. (2004). Opioid-induced hyperalgesia and opioid rotation. *Journal of Pain & Palliative Care Pharmacology, 18*(3), 75–79.

Institute for Clinical Systems Improvement. (2008). *Assessment and management of chronic pain.* Bloomington, MN: Institute for Clinical Systems Improvement.

Løvlie, R., Daly, A. K., Matre, G. E., Molven, A., & Steen, V. M. (2001). Polymorphisms in CYP2D6 duplication-negative individuals with the ultrarapid metabolizer phenotype: A role for the CYP2D6*35 allele in ultrarapid metabolism? *Pharmacogenetics, 11*(1), 45–55.

McCoy, A. (n.d.). *Opium history up to 1858 AD.* Retrieved from http:// opioids.com/opium/history/index

Pasternak, G. W. (2004). Multiple opiate receptors: Déjà vu all over again. *Neuropharmacology, 47*(Suppl. 1), 312–323.

The plant of joy: A brief history of opium. (n.d.). Retrieved from http://www .opiates.net/

Snyder, S., & Pasternak, G. (2003). Historical review: Opioid receptors. *Trends in Pharmacological Sciences, 24*(4), 198–205.

Stanos S., Fishbain, D., & Fishman, S. (2009). Pain management with opioid analgesics: Balancing risk and benefit. *Physical Medicine & Rehabilitation, 88*(3, Suppl. 2), S69–S99.

5

Coanalgesics for Additive Pain Relief

COANALGESICS FOR CHRONIC PAIN

Coanalgesics are a varied group of medications that can provide additive pain relief when they are added to nonsteroidal anti-inflammatory drugs (NSAIDs) or opioids (American Pain Society [APS], 2008). They can have independent analgesic activity for some painful complaints, and they can counteract select adverse effects of analgesics (APS, 2008). This group of medications was developed to treat a wide variety of conditions, such as seizures or muscle spasms, and was originally intended for symptom control of the various conditions. However, in many cases, patients reported pain relief when these medications were prescribed for them, leading health care providers to consider their additional application for pain relief.

Medications that are considered to be coanalgesic for pain management include the following:

- Antidepressants
- Anticonvulsants
- Muscle relaxants
- Topical agents
- Cannabinoids
- *N*-methyl-D-aspartate (NMDA) receptor blockers
- Alpha-2 adrenergic agonists
- Benzodiazepines

■ Antispasmodic agents
■ Stimulants (APS, 2008)

Although these medications were not developed for pain control, they have been used for adjunct pain relief and are found to be effective. For some medications, such as gabapentin, pregabalin, and duloxetine, the unapproved use for pain management became so prevalent that the manufacturers sought and received Food and Drug Administration (FDA) approval for the pain management indication. Many patients with neuropathic pain benefit greatly from the addition of one or more of these agents to help decrease pain. Because many patients with chronic pain are depressed, the use of antidepressants has improved the quality of pain relief and enhanced sleep for many of these patients.

When the World Health Organization (WHO) ladder was developed with medication choices for pain management (see Chapter 3), the focus was on dividing different types of opioid medications. However, the ladder also includes adjuvant medications, or coanalgesics, on each step of the ladder. The broad classes of these medications are listed on the ladder steps, but no specific medications are listed (Dalton & Youngblood, 2000).

Trying to group these medications into a single class, coanalgesics, is difficult. They all have such different mechanisms of action and application. These medications can enhance the effect of opioids or other medication that are being used for pain relief, or they can stand alone as single agent pain relievers (APS, 2008). Some of the benefits of using these medications include the following:

■ Enhance pain relief
■ Allow lower doses of opioids (opioid sparing effect)
■ Manage refractory pain
■ Reduce side effects of opioids related to opioid sparing (APS, 2008)

Commonly used coanalgesics include the following:

■ acetaminophen
■ ibuprofen or naproxen
■ celecoxib
■ gabapentin and pregabalin

- duloxetine
- Topical lidocaine and capsaicin
- cyclobenzaprine, carisoprodol, metaxalone
- diazepam, alprazolam (APS, 2008)

No matter which medication is selected or combined with another pain medication, each patient's comorbidities and related treatments need to be assessed and evaluated before adding a new medication to the pain management medication regimen. The following sections of the chapter will discuss different classes of coanalgesic that can be used for additional pain relief.

ANTIDEPRESSANT MEDICATIONS

Antidepressant medications are classed into several different types, which include the following:

- Tricyclic
- Selective serotonin reuptake inhibitors (SSRI)
- Selective serotonin norepinephrine reuptake inhibitors (SSNRI)

Antidepressant medications have several different mechanisms of action. The tricyclic antidepressants (TCAs; see Table 5.1), such as amitriptyline, inhibit presynaptic uptake of norepinephrine and serotonin, as do the SSNRIs, such as duloxetine. Other less studied actions for TCAs include a mild opioid action at the mu binding sites, sodium and calcium channel blockade, NMDA site antagonism, and adenosine activity (Lynch & Watson, 2006). The SSRI medications, such as fluoxetine, inhibit serotonin at the presynaptic junction site (American Society of Pain Management Nurses [ASPMN], 2009). The effect of this inhibition decreases the ability of the pain stimulus to be transmitted higher up the central nervous system. These medications are most commonly used as adjunct medication for neuropathic-type pain, such as postherpetic neuralgia, painful diabetic neuropathies, and neuropathic syndromes (Lynch & Watson, 2006). They are also a good adjunct in patients with cancer and neuropathic pain when opioids have provided suboptimal pain relief (APS, 2008).

Table 5.1 ■ *Tricyclic Antidepressants*

Common TCAs	Starting Dose	Effective Dose
amitriptyline (Elavil)	10–25 mg hs	50–150 mg hs
desipramine (Norpramin)	10–25 mg hs	50–150 mg hs
nortriptyline (Pamelor)	10–25 mg hs	50–150 mg hs

Abbreviations: hs, at bedtime; TCAs, tricyclic antidepressants.
Source: From American Pain Society, 2008.

Tricyclic Antidepressants

The TCAs were, at one time, considered to be the first line for treating neuropathic pain, such as postherpetic neuralgia or postmastectomy pain syndromes. Currently, they have fallen to lower down on the option list as newer and better medications with fewer side effects have been developed. They are not recommended for older patients, because they have the potential for orthostatic hypotension (American Geriatric Society [AGS], 2009).

The starting doses are low and start at 10–25 mg titrated up to 150 mg per day (APS, 2008; Wallace & Staats, 2005). Escalating to higher doses in an effort to obtain an additive effect for pain relief should take place every 3–7 days (Chen, Lamer, Rho, Marshall, Sitzman, Ghazi & Brewer, 2004). The pain management doses are lower than the antidepressant doses of 150–30 mg per day. Of note, the pain relief action of these medications is independent of any effect on mood (Lynch & Watson, 2006).

A meta-analysis of the TCA medications indicates that TCAs are effective for use in treating neuropathic pain (APS, 2003). Elavil (amitriptyline) is the best known and most studied among the TCAs (APS, 2003). It is also a primary recommendation for the treatment of fibromyalgia pain (D'Arcy & McCarberg, 2005). Analgesic response is usually seen within 5–7 days (APS, 2008). Adverse effects for TCAS include:

■ Sedation
■ Dry mouth
■ Constipation

- Urinary retention
- Orthostatic hypotension
- Anticholinergic side effects
- Caution in patients with heart disease, symptomatic prostatic hypertrophy, neurogenic bladder, dementia, or narrow angle glaucoma
- Increased suicide behavior in young adults (Institute for Clinical System Improvement [ICSI], 2007)

These side effects make the medications undesirable for use in the elderly population of patients, especially when they are used in combination with opioid analgesics.

Additionally, TCAs can increase the risk of cardiac arrhythmias in patients with underlying conduction abnormalities. Caution is advised with the use of desipramine in children because of anecdotal reports of sudden death (APS, 2003). Although these drugs are cheap and readily available, they do have some very significant adverse effects. At the opposite end of the spectrum, they also have the best profile for use in treating neuropathic pain conditions. However, each patient being considered for TCAs should have a thorough assessment for any risk factors, such as cardiac conduction abnormalities. When starting TCA therapy, the current recommendation is to screen all patients older than 40 years with an electrocardiogram (ECG) to evaluate the patients for conduction abnormalities (APS, 2008).

The TCA medications are not recommended for use in elderly patients, because of the high incidence of undesirable side effects and the potential for increased fall risk related to early morning orthostatic hypotension (AGS, 2002, 2009; Lynch & Watson, 2006). The biggest benefits of using TCAs for pain relief are improved sleep (Wilson, Caplan, Connis, Gilbert, Grigsby, Haddox, Simon, 1997) and the relief of neuropathic pain—pain that is described by patients as burning, shooting, or painful numbness.

When caring for a patient who is taking TCAs as adjuvant pain medication, health care providers should be aware of the potential for early morning orthostatic hypotension and caution the patient to sit on the side of the bed before trying to stand. Some patients complain of sleepiness with these medications and, if this is problematic, the patient should be instructed to take the medication earlier in the evening rather than at bedtime to decrease the early morning sedation that can be experienced. For elderly men, urinary retention can be problematic and urinary status should be carefully checked. For the dry mouth associated with TCA use, hard candies or gum can ease the dry feeling.

Patients should always be told the rationale for prescribing an antidepressant medication for pain, so they are comfortable with taking the medication. The onset of analgesic effect may take up to 2 weeks, and patients should be encouraged to extend a trial of these medications to this period to see if analgesia occurs.

SELECTIVE SEROTONIN REUPTAKE INHIBITORS

Of all three groups of antidepressants, the SSRI group (see Table 5.2) has the poorest profile for pain relief (APS, 2006). When compared with placebo, these medications did not have any significant advantage for pain relief. Given the lack of efficacy for pain relief in these medications and the profile of side effects, sexual dysfunction, anxiety, sleep disorder, and headache, the SSRIs are not medications that should be given unless there is a specific indication for use. The recommended use for this group of medications is for patients who have concurrent depression, anxiety, or insomnia (APS, 2008).

Table 5.2 ■ *Selective Serotonin Reuptake Inhibitors*

Common SSRIs	Starting Dose	Effective Dose
paroxetine (Paxil)	10–20 mg daily	20–40 mg daily
citalopram (Celexa)	10–20 mg daily	20–40 mg daily

Source: From American Pain Society, 2008.

SELECTIVE SEROTONIN AND NOREPINEPHRINE REUPTAKE INHIBITORS

The pain relief mechanism of the SSNRI group (see Table 5.3) of antidepressants is the inhibition of serotonin and norepinephrine at therapeutic doses. The SNRI medications do not have the same anticholinergic side effect profile as the TCA medications. They are effective for various neuropathic pain conditions, such as diabetic neuropathy, postherpetic neuralgia, and atypical facial pain (Lynch & Watson, 2006). Venlafaxine has shown an effect on hyperalgesia and allodynia—preventing the occurrence and decreasing the pain (Wallace & Staats, 2005; APS, 2008). Effective doses for venlafaxine for pain relief range from 150 mg to 225 mg, with a starting dose of 37.5 mg.

Duloxetine has received FDA approval for treating painful diabetic neuropathy (PDN). For duloxetine, the starting dose of 20 mg per day may decrease the incidence of side effects, with pain relief experienced at a dose range from 60 mg per day to 120 mg per day. Careful titration of the medications and slow dose increases will help decrease some of the side effects, such as somnolence, nausea, and sweating. There have been no identified increased cardiovascular risks associated with the use of duloxetine (APS, 2008).

There are some drawbacks with both venlafaxine and duloxetine. There is an increased risk of suicidal ideation and behavior in children and adolescents with major depressive disorders, and venlafaxine and duloxetine are not approved for pediatric patients. Care should also be taken with patients who have liver disease or use alcohol consistently (Cymbalta package insert, prescribing information, available

Table 5.3 ■ *Serotonin and Norepinephrine Reuptake Inhibitors*

Common SNRIs	*Starting Dose*	*Effective Dose*
venlafaxine (Effexor)	37.5 mg daily	150–225 mg daily
duloxetine (Cymbalta)	20 mg daily	60 mg daily

Source: From American Pain Society, 2008.

at http://www.PrescribingReference.com). There is also the potential for the development of sick serotonin syndrome, which occurs when patients taking SNRI medications take other medications that affect serotonin production, such as SSRI medications.

Cardiac changes, such as atrioventricular (AV) block and increases in blood pressure, are possible (Lynch & Watson, 2006). Five percent of patients treated with venlafaxine developed changes on ECG (APS, 2008). As a result, patients who are taking venlafaxine who also have diabetes mellitus, hypertension, or hypercholesterolemia, or are currently smoking should have ECG monitoring while on the antidepressant medication (APS, 2008). Patients who are taking these medications for adjunct pain relief should have regular blood pressure screenings and should be assessed regularly for any signs of cardiac changes. Careful dose tapering should take place when these medications are being discontinued to avoid discontinuation syndrome, insomnia, lethargy, diarrhea, nausea, dizziness, or paresthesia (APS, 2008).

The newest SSNRI medication with a pain indication is milnacipran (Savella). It is used to treat the centrally amplified pain of fibromyalgia. The serotonin component of the medication is thought to affect depression, although the norepinephrine component is thought to improve chronic pain. In more than 2,000 patients, milnacipran at both 100 and 200 mg per day doses was shown to be superior to placebo for controlling the pain of fibromyalgia. It is 85% bioavailable.

As with other medications in this class, monoamine oxidase (MAO) inhibitors are contraindicated, as is tryptophan. Additional interaction may occur with amphetamines, aspirin, clonidine, digoxin, tramadol, hypertension medication, triptans used for migraines, NSAIDs, lithium, epinephrine, furazolidone, and linezolid (Gold Standard website, available at http://www.bing.com/health/article/goldstandard). Doses should be titrated up carefully, starting with 12.5 mg by mouth per day, then 12.5 mg twice per day on days 2–3, then 25 mg twice per day on days 4–7, and thereafter 50 mg twice per day. Maximum dose is 200 mg per day. Side effects are similar to those of other medications in this class.

ANTICONVULSANT MEDICATIONS

Anticonvulsants (see Table 5.4), such as gabapentin, pregabalin, carbamazepine, topiramate, and phenytoin, are commonly used to treat many types of neuropathic pain, including postherpetic neuralgia, PDN, and trigeminal neuralgia (APS, 2006). The original premise for use of these medications for neuropathic pain management was that if these medications could control the erratic neuronal firing or seizures, they might be applied to controlling neuronal discharge from pain stimuli. Research has shown that this is essentially true and that one of the primary mechanisms of these medications is to reduce neuronal excitability and spontaneous firing of cortical neurons (APS, 2008). When applied to pain management, these drugs decrease the neuronal firing after nerve damage, treat neuropathic pain, and decrease neuronal sensitization (APS, 2008).

Gabapentin is one of the medications used to treat a multitude of neuropathic pain syndromes, but it is particularly effective with postherpetic neuralgia, diabetic neuropathy, phantom limb pain, Guillain-Barré syndrome, neuropathic cancer pain, and acute and chronic spinal cord injury (APS, 2008; ICSI, 2007). Syndromes that do not respond to gabapentin are HIV-related neuropathy and painful peripheral chemotherapy-induced neuropathies (APS, 2008).

Both gabapentin and pregabalin act by blocking neuronal calcium channels, the alpha 2-delta subunit specifically, thereby reducing the release of glutamate, norepinephrine, and substance P (APS, 2008). Because the drugs are renally excreted, dose reductions are advised for

Table 5.4 ■ *Anticonvulsant Medications*

Commonly Used Anticonvulsants	Starting Dose	Effective Dose
gabapentin (Neurontin)	100–300 mg hs	300–1,200 mg tid
pregabalin (Lyrica)	150 mg daily	300–600 mg daily
carbamazepine (Tegretol)	100–200 mg daily	300–800 mg bid
topiramate (Topamax)	25 mg daily	100–200 mg bid
phenytoin (Dilantin)	300 mg hs	100–150 mg tid

Abbreviations: bid, twice daily; hs, at bedtime; tid, three times a day.

patients with renal impairment. The one drawback to gabapentin is the length of time needed to reach effective dose strength because it is only 10% bioavailable. Because medication response is patient-dependent, it may takes weeks or months to reach a dose of gabapentin that will provide pain relief. Pregabalin, as an alternate option, can provide a faster response for pain relief because it is 90% bioavailable, and therapeutic doses can be given earlier in the treatment.

The older anticonvulsants, such as phenytoin (Dilantin), have not been studied for pain relief to the extent that the newer gabapentin medications have and, thus, only weak evidence is available for their use as coanalgesic medications for pain. There is a need for further research data on these medications. One early meta-analysis (APS, 2008) on four anticonvulsants, phenytoin, carbamazepine, clonazepam, and valproate, determined that these anticonvulsants were effective for relieving the pain of trigeminal neuralgia, diabetic neuropathy, and migraine prophylaxis. Given the high profile for serious adverse side effects, the new gabapentin medications are indicated as a first-line choice for treating neuropathic pain (APS, 2008).

One of the major drawbacks to anticonvulsant medication use for pain management is their high profile for adverse side effects. These include the following:

- Somnolence
- Dizziness
- Fatigue
- Nausea
- Edema
- Weight gain
- Stevens-Johnson syndrome
- Increased risk of suicidal behavior or ideation
- Aplastic anemia and agranulocytosis (ICSI, 2007)

The serious nature of the adverse side effects of this class of medications make it imperative that when starting these medications, a full baseline history is taken from the patient. Careful monitoring is required, and patients should be instructed to report the occurrence and severity of any adverse effect experienced.

TOPICAL ANALGESICS

■ *Lidocaine 5% Patch (Lidoderm)*

When the patient has a specific tender point or has an area of pain that is limited, it is tempting to use a type of pain relief that will affect only the painful area. The lidocaine patch is a soft flannel–backed patch with 5% lidocaine that can be applied over the painful area. It has an indication for use with postherpetic neuralgia and has been studied in painful diabetic neuropathy, complex regional pain syndrome, postmastectomy pain, and HIV-related neuropathy (APS, 2008).

The patch is designed to be used for 12 hours on and 12 hours off, although patients have worn the patch for 24 hours with no ill effects (APS, 2008; D'Arcy, 2007). The maximum dose of Lidoderm is up to three patches at one time. The patches should be replaced daily and placed only on intact skin. Active serum levels of lidocaine with patch use are minimal (APS,2008). Patients tolerate this type of therapy very well, and, because it is noninvasive, if the patient does not like the feeling of the patch or effect, the patch can be easily removed. The one side effect from the Lidoderm patch that has been reported is skin irritation at the site of patch application.

■ *Capsaicin Cream (Zostrix)*

This topical cream that can reduce the secretion of substance P at peripheral nerve ending is derived from hot peppers and is called capsaicin. It is sold over the counter in two different strengths as a generic brand or Zostrix cream. The neuropathic conditions for which this cream has been most helpful include postmastectomy pain, other peripheral neuropathic conditions, and neck and arthritis pain (APS, 2008).

When the cream is applied, it causes a burning sensation in the application area. Patients should be warned to expect the sensation. Gloves should be used to apply the cream and other parts of the body, such as the eyes, should not be touched until all the cream is removed from the hands. Use of this technique requires a dedicated patient who is willing to persevere and apply the cream three to four times per day for 2 weeks to see if there is any analgesic benefit.

The newest use of capsaicin is a concentrated 8% patch (Qutenza) for postherpetic neuralgia that needs to have a local anesthetic applied at the site of patch placement prior to the placement. The patch is left in place for 1 hour, and then removed. This is a technique that requires a health care provider for application. Studies have shown improved pain relief with patch applications and extended effect with sustained pain relief for up to 12 weeks. Certainly, this not a common use for capsaicin, but for the select few who need it, the technique can provide improved pain relief (Dworkin et al., 2010).

Targeted Analgesic-Diclofenac Epolamine Patch (Flector)

The Flector Patch is a nonselective NSAID patch that is applied directly over the site of the pain on intact skin. It is especially useful for strains and sprains. The recommended dose is one patch to the affected area twice daily (*Nursing 2010 Drug Handbook*, 2009). Because this is a new use for NSAIDs, the research support is limited, and data on systemic absorption are open to change when clinical usage increases. Currently, the medication has the same black box warning as all nonselective NSAIDs.

There are compounded gels and over-the-counter NSAID gel and liquid formulations as well. These can be very effective if used as directed in the prescribed area. However, with continued use and application over large areas, there is an increased potential for systemic absorption. Patients are advised to use the application card supplied with the medication and to wear gloves when applying the gel (*Nursing 2010 Drug Handbook*, 2009).

MUSCLE RELAXANTS

Muscle relaxants are a good addition to a pain regimen for low back pain, where muscle spasms occur regularly. They are also useful for conditions such as fibromyalgia, where cyclobenzaprine is considered a first-line option (APS, 2005; D'Arcy & McCarberg, 2005). The group of medications generically called skeletal muscle relaxants (see Table 5.5) consists of several different groups of medications: benzodiazepines, sedatives, antihistamines, and other centrally acting medications (APS, 2008).

Table 5.5 ■ *Skeletal Muscle Relaxants*

Commonly Used Muscle Relaxants	Starting Dose	Effective Dose
cyclobenzaprine (Flexeril)	5 mg tid	10–20 mg tid
carisoprodol (Soma)	350 mg hs-tid	350 mg tid-qid
orphenadrine (Norflex)	100 mg bid	100 mg bid
tizanidine (Zanaflex)	2 mg hs	variable
metaxalone (Skelaxin)	400 mg tid-qid	800 mg tid-qid
methocarbamol (Robaxin)	500 mg qid	500–750 mg qid
Other:		
antispasmodic—baclofen	5 mg tid	10–20 mg tid
benzodiazepine—diazepam	1 mg bid	2–10 mg bid-qid

Abbreviations: bid, twice daily; hs, at bedtime; tid, three times a day; qid, four times a day.
Source: From American Pain Society, 2008.

Although there is no indication that these medications relax skeletal muscles, they are commonly used for spasm and muscle tightness (APS, 2008). After 1–2 weeks, the action of the medication shifts to a central activity rather than skeletal muscle activity (APS, 2008). The most common side effect of this group of medications is sedation. If they are being used concomitantly with an opioid analgesics, the sedative effect is cumulative. There is the potential for abuse in patients who are predisposed to this problem, so intermittent or short-term use is advised.

OTHER COANALGESICS

There are various other medications that can be used as coanalgesics— ranging from cannabinoids and dronabinol that are recommended for neuropathic pain from multiple sclerosis to NMDA receptor blockers, ketamine, dextromethorphan, and amantadine that are used for centrally mediated neuropathic pain and hyperalgesia. These agents are not recommended for first- or second-line use, but, rather, for patients in whom all other attempts at pain relief have failed. They have a high profile for such little research support and lean more on anecdotal and single study support.

These medications also have a high profile for significant adverse side effects. Dronabinol use can cause cognitive impairment, psychosis, and sedation (APS, 2008).

The NMDA receptor blockers have significant adverse side effects as well. Ketamine can cause hallucinations, memory problems, and abuse potential, and amantadine and dextromethorphan have side effects, such as dizziness, insomnia, and nausea (*Nursing 2010 Drug Handbook*, 2009).

When considering using a coanalgesic, the health care provider needs to fully assess the patient and consider all the comorbidities and potential drug–drug interactions. The use of these medications is highly individual, and doses may vary according to the patient's ability to tolerate the medications. Starting a lower doses and escalating slowly can help reduce the seriousness of the side effects. Because analgesic effect can take time to become apparent, patients should be encouraged to use these medications for at least 2 weeks before deciding they are not effective for pain relief.

June is a 57-year-old patient who has had diabetes for 10 years. She also has hypertension, hypercholesterolemia, and depression. Over the past 10 years, she has been on various diabetic agents but cannot keep her hemoglobin A1C levels at the required level. She does not exercise and has been gaining weight steadily. She has recently reported some changes in sensation in her feet. She reports that the pain is burning and shooting in nature and it worsens at night. For the pain, she is taking Oxycontin 20 mg twice a day and using Percocet for breakthrough pain. She uses Ambien for sleep. When you ask her about her, pain she tells you, "The pain just started by itself. First, there was this numb feeling in my feet. I noticed I kept running into things. Then the burning pain started. It never really gets better, but during the day I can tolerate it better. It ranges from pain intensity of 5/10–8/10 at night. The other day I looked down and I had an open area on my foot that I didn't even know was here. Is there something I can do to make this pain better?"

You diagnose June with painful diabetic neuropathy (PDN). Even if she can get her A1C levels down, the pain will continue at some level. Aside from the diabetes, hypertension, and hypercholesterolemia medications, you will need to include some medications for pain in addition to the opioids, which do not seem to be affecting the pain intensity.

Questions to Consider

1. What type of coanalgesics are recommended for neuropathic pain like June's?
2. What effect will June's comorbidities have on your medication choices?
3. Could you stop the opioids and still get a good pain relief with one or more of the coanalgesic medications?
4. Will June's pain ever fully resolve?
5. What coanalgesics are not recommended for a patient like June?

REFERENCES

American Geriatrics Society. (2002). The management of persistent pain in older persons. *Journal of the American Geriatrics Society, 50,* S205–S224.

American Geriatrics Society. (2009). The management of persistent pain in older persons. *Journal of the American Geriatrics Society, 50,* S205–S224.

American Pain Society. (2006). *Pain control in the primary care setting.* Glenview, IL: Author.

American Pain Society. (2008). *Principles of analgesic use in the treatment of acute and cancer pain.* Glenview, IL: Author.

American Society of Pain Management Nurses. (2009). *Core curriculum for pain management nursing.* Philadelphia, PA: W.B. Saunders.

Chen, H., Lamer, T. J., Rho, R. H., Marshall, K. A., Sitzman, B. T., Ghazi, S. M., & Brewer R. (2004). Contemporary management of neuropathic pain for the primary care physician. *Mayo Clinic Proceedings, 79*(12), 1533–1545.

Dalton, J. A., & Youngblood, R. (2000). Clinical application of the world health organization analgesic ladder. *Journal of IV Nursing, 23*(2), 118–124.

D'Arcy, Y. (2007). *Pain management: Evidence-based tools and techniques for nursing professionals.* Marblehead, MA: HCPro.

D'Arcy, Y., & McCarberg, B. (2005). New fibromyalgia pain management recommendations. *The Journal for Nurse Practitioners, 4,* 218–225.

Dworkin, R. H., O'Connor, A. B., Audette, J., Baron, R., Gourlay, G. K., Haanpää, M. L., et al. (2010, March). [Review]. *Mayo Clinic Proceedings, 85*(Suppl. 3), S3–14.

Institute for Clinical System Improvement. (2008). *Assessment and management of chronic pain.* Retrieved from http://www.guideline.gov

Lynch, M., & Watson, C. (2006). The pharmacotherapy of chronic pain: A review. *Pain Research & Management: The Journal of the Canadian Pain Society, 11*(1), 11–38.

Nursing 2010 Drug Handbook. (2009). Philadelphia, PA: Wolters Kluwer/ Lippincott Williams & Wilkins.

Wallace, M., & Staats, P. (2005). *Pain medicine & management.* New York, NY: McGraw-Hill.

Wilson, P., Caplan, R., Connis, R., Gilbert, H., Grigsby, E., Haddox D., . . . Simon, D. (1997). Practice guidelines for chronic pain management: A report by the American Society of Anesthesiologists Task Force on Pain Management, Chronic Pain Section. *Anesthesiology, 86*(4), 995–1004.

ADDITIONAL RESOURCES

American Society of Pain Management Nurses. (2002). *Core curriculum for pain management nursing.* Philadelphia, PA: W.B. Saunders.

6

Complementary and Integrative Therapies for Pain Management

OVERVIEW

Patients like to have some control over the way their pain is treated, and many of them like and are interested in using techniques that are called *alternative, integrated, integrative* or *complementary.* This does not mean that they forego standard medical care, but that they add these additional treatment options into their pain relief regimen. Patients can use hot or cold therapy, yoga, or walking to help stay in shape and increase their ability to function. Patients like to have a holistic approach to treating pain that recognizes not only the physical pain but includes the mantel and emotional aspects. In many cases the patients do not have to forego standard medical treatment but can add a more comprehensive approach adding in integrative techniques that can enhance pain relief.

Some of the advantages of these integrative techniques include the following:

■ Low or no cost
■ Patients can control many of the options
■ Readily available and many do not require a prescription

Many patients have a favorite, tried and true pain relief measure they use before they consider trying to find help for a pain problem. Other patients are focused on wellness and have techniques they use to relieve stress, such as yoga or relaxation, that can also be very beneficial for pain relief. Patients who have arthritis or a muscle strain or sprain

121

may try a mild analgesic they may have in their medicine chest, along with a little light exercise or heat or ice to relieve the pain. Topical creams, such as Ben Gay or Icy Hot, are very popular with older patients who have this type of pain complaint (Khatta, 2007).

Because these types of treatments are available over the counter, seen on television, or recommended by word of mouth for effectiveness, there is little research base that recommends one treatment option over the other. Looking for the research base in this area of medicine can be confusing to say the least because the research may be very broad and patient outcomes may not be clearly identified. With the increased popularity of these techniques more research studies and outcomes are being developed.

Because of the confusing research and outcomes information, the National Institutes of Health (NIH) is studying the use of alternative treatments and has a group called the National Center for Complementary and Alternative Medicine (NCCAM, 2004). The goal of this group of researchers is to review all the literature support and come to some recommendations about how effective and safe these treatments are. Because there is such a big interest in using organic substances, herbal remedies, and vitamin supplements for promoting health and alleviating some forms of pain, such as arthritis, this group has started a review of the common herbs and supplements being used to treat common conditions. Other areas of study include energy therapies and treatments such as chiropractic manipulation and acupuncture.

The general term to refer to these methods has been shortened to complementary and alternative medicine (CAM). CAM is defined as "a group of diverse medical and health care systems, practices, and products not presently considered to be a part of conventional medicine" (American Pain Society [APS], 2006). These techniques are meant to supplement and not replace standard medical therapies and medication.

Most patients are a bit shy about informing their health care practitioner about extra supplements and home remedies they are using. They feel the health care provider may make them feel uncomfortable about trying something that has not been prescribed for the condition. Many patients will openly tell the health care staff about their special supplements and herbal remedies if they are asked in a nonjudgmental way. Because some of these compounds can have a drug–drug interaction with the medication, it is important for the health care provider to ask questions about these types of remedies and supplements; therefore, a full medication/supplement history is taken. Patients may not even consider this information important, but for the health care provider it can be an integral piece of the patient's history.

CAM techniques are attractive options for most patients. They do not require a prescription, the patient controls the use, and side effects are not common. Most medications for chronic pain can have side effects, such as constipation, sedation, or dizziness, to name a few. Cost can also be a factor. Aside from supplements and herbal remedies, there is little to no cost for relaxation, biofeedback, or imagery.

Where do the patients get information about CAM therapies? Many publications, such as women's magazines and the American Association of Retired Persons magazine, have articles on yoga, pool therapy, or relaxation for health and stress management. Patients are also very Internet savvy. They can search websites for information about any therapy or supplement of interest to them. Older patients are no exception. They can find information as easily as younger patients and may be willing to try something that seems to offer a quick, easy way to relieve pain (APS, 2002). Health care providers should never underestimate the power of word of mouth. Something discussed at the bridge game last evening may show up in the examining room today. Senior Citizen Centers also provide educational offerings that can include information on different types of CAM therapies.

Because many Americans are open to using CAM therapies to help relieve pain, practitioners of various therapies, such as yoga or acupuncture, have become common. Patients should be encouraged to ask these practitioners about their training and expertise in the technique they are providing. There are schools for massage and certificates for practitioners, such as Reiki, that are given to those who have completed the classes required to practice the technique. For a patient to go to an acupuncturist with little or no training or expertise, for example, may be more harmful than helpful.

In a 1997 survey, Americans reported that they made 629 million visits to CAM practitioners. In other parts of the world about 20% to 70% of all patients use CAM therapies. Primary care practitioners responded that they do not ask patients about the use of CAM therapies. Only 40% of patients volunteer information on their use of CAM therapies. In a 2002 survey, the most common conditions for which patients used CAM to help relieve pain were:

- Back pain
- Neck pain
- Joint pain
- Arthritis
- Headache (NCCAM, 2002; Pierce, 2009).

There can be no doubt that many patients, both old and young, find CAM modalities helpful for pain relief.

TYPES OF CAM THERAPIES

Chronic pain is one of the primary reasons that patients try CAM therapies. Patients look for ways to relieve not only the daily pain but the anxiety and uncertainty that the pain produces. Many of the techniques are minimally invasive, such as acupuncture, or noninvasive, such as the energy therapies of Reiki or therapeutic touch (TT). Because many patients are attracted to this type of therapy, incorporating it into the plan of care can help track outcomes and determine benefit. Because the use of these therapeutics is controversial and research is limited, it is helpful to monitor the benefit of these therapies when they are added to a plan of care.

Many terms are applied to CAM therapies. Terms have changed through the years and some common terms are listed below. Currently, *integrative* is the term most often used with this category of therapeutic options.

Complementary: Techniques or additional therapies that are used in conjunction with recognized mainstream medical practices; for example, when music or relaxation is used with medication for low back pain.

Alternative: This term means foregoing recognized medical therapy and using other treatments for a condition; for example, when vitamin supplements, magnets and/or imagery is used in place of traditional cancer treatments.

Integrative: A term coined by CAM practitioners to indicate the combined use of pharmacotherapy and nonpharmacologic methods for medical treatment. This term was first used by Dr. Andrew Weil and is the most common term applied to CAM therapies at this time. (NCCAM, 2004)

There are many different types of CAM therapies that are available for treating pain. Some are very simple to use, such as hot or cold therapy. Others, such as biofeedback, require patients to be educated about using the technique. Still others, such as TT, require a trained practitioner to administer them.

The four main areas or types of CAM as defined by the NCCAM are:

- **Body-based therapies,** such as hot and cold therapy, massage, yoga, exercise, and acupuncture
- **Cognitive behavioral approaches** or mind–body work, such as relaxation, biofeedback, meditation, distraction, and imagery
- **Energy medicine**, including Reiki, Healing Touch, and TT
- **Nutritional approaches** that incorporate the use of diet, herbs and vitamin supplements

Body-Based Therapies
Hot and Cold Therapy

Hot and cold applications are common home remedies. Patients are comfortable with the idea of using a heating pad for back pain or applying a cold pack for a minor muscle injury. Every household has an assortment of heating pads, ice packs, and the newer versions of microwave heating pads and wraps. Most patients find more comfort in heat and prefer it over cold packs. As for research support, a Cochrane report with low back pain patients indicates the therapies have limited support (French, Cameron, Walker, Reggars, Esterman, 2006). However, additional information indicates that a heat wrap can increase functionality in patients with low back pain (French, 2006).

The benefit of using a heating pad or hot pack can increase circulation to the affected area, decrease stiffness, reduce pain, and relieve muscle spasms (American Society of Pain Management Nurses [ASPMN], 2010). When using heat, patients should be cautioned to:

- Use it for short periods of time.
- Monitor use carefully over areas of decreased circulation to avoid burns.
- Avoid placing it over areas where mentholated creams have been used, which can increase the potential for skin damage.
- Heat should never be placed over a patch delivering medications such as fentanyl, medications for hypertension, or smoking cessation patches. The heat over these patches will increase the delivery of the medication to the patients and put them at risk for overdose. (Taken from D'Arcy, 2010)

Ice baths, cold packs, or ice massage are helpful for decreasing the pain minor injuries, low back pain, and muscle spasms (ASPMN, 2010). Many older patients refuse to try cold applications although it can be helpful for pain relief. The cold applications work by:

- Decreased nerve conduction
- Cutaneous counterirritation
- Vasoconstriction
- Muscle relaxation
- Reduction of local and systemic metabolic activity (ASPMN, 2010)

To improve the use of hot and cold therapy and avoid tissue damage, they should be used for intermittent short periods of time only. Patients with cardiovascular disease and diabetes, should take care to monitor the application sites for skin damage.

A common approach used by health care providers for patients with a minor ache or sprain is RICE therapy:

- **R**est
- **I**ce
- **C**ompression
- **E**levation (Berry, Covington, Dahl, Katz, Miaskowski, 2006)

For patients with chronic pain, this technique may be less useful; during exacerbation of musculoskeletal pain, however, it may provide some added relief.

Acupuncture

Acupuncture is one of the oldest CAM therapies. It originated in China where it balanced the yin and yang or energy of life forces (ASPMN, 2010). The Chinese believe that balancing the life energies creates a flow of energy called Chi or QI life energy forces along meridians located in the body (Weintraub, Mamtani, & Micozzi, 2008). If the flow of energy is blocked, weak, or in a state of imbalance, an illness or pain will occur (Khatta, 2007). Acupuncture restores balance to the body and open up the blocked chakras or energy blockages.

Acupuncture has several different variations in practice, depending on the part of the world where the practice originates. The classic approach is Chinese, and there are medical artifacts from history that indicate that acupuncture was used as a regular part of Chinese medicine for many centuries.

When acupuncture is performed, thin needles are inserted through the skin into predetermined points designed to release the blocked energy (ASPMN, 2010; Dillard & Knapp, 2005; NCCAM, 2004). The needles are manipulated by hand or electrically stimulated releasing neurotransmitters that can decrease pain (Dillard & Knapp, 2005).

Conditions for which acupuncture has been used include:

- Fibromyalgia
- Osteoarthritis
- Labor pain
- Low back pain, nausea associated with chemotherapy and pregnancy (Weintraub, Mamatani, Micozzi, 2008)
- Dental pain (APS, 2005; Dillard & Knapp, 2005)

In a study of 570 patients with osteoarthritis receiving acupuncture, the patients in the study had improvements in function and decreased pain levels (Khatta, 2007). In a review of acupunture used for relief of low back pain, the outcome proved the treatment to be better than sham or no treatment for pain relief and improved function, but there was a recommendation for more research on the technique (Furlan, Brosseau, Imamura, Irvin, 2002). For low back pain, acupuncture was found to be more effective than sham acupuncture.

Massage

NIH and NCCAM define massage as pressing, rubbing, and otherwise manipulating muscles and soft tissue in the body (NCCAM, 2004). Massage can take several different forms, with deep tissue massage or a lighter technique. Aromatherapy can be combined with massage to make the experience more relaxing. Massage increases oxygenation and blood flow to the area which lengthens and relaxes the muscles. (NCCAM, 2004). Compared with other noninvasive interventions, massage can produce effective pain relief. Conditions for which massage has been found to be helpful are:

- Stress management and comfort
- Pain management
- Improving mobility and movement
- Edema
- Part of a physical therapy regimen (Weintraub et al., 2008)
- The popularity of massage is increasing with many patients requesting massage therapy from their physicians and if not covered by insurance about 90% of the patients for the treatment out of pocket (Weintraub et al., 2008)

Chiropractic

Chiropractic treatment or adjustments consist of spinal manipulation and other techniques to align the body to reduce pain. About 90% of all patients who are referred to chiropractic treatment are seen for musculoskeletal pain; back, neck and headache pain (Weintraub et al., 2008). The findings on using chiropractic for pain relief are mixed. For low back pain, however, there is good evidence that chiropractic therapy is effective for chronic or subacute low back pain.

Other Types of Body-Based Therapies

Other forms of body-based therapies are not a well supported by research. These therapies include:

- Magnets
- Copper bracelets

However, those that do have support can be useful to help relieve pain. Physical therapy has benefit for those patients who are able to comply with the physical demands. The benefit of physical therapy is to recondition a weakened patient, improve mood, reduce pain and maintain mobility while increasing overall functionality (APS, 2002; Bruckenthal & D'Arcy, 2007). For low back pain, exercise has good evidence to support it for pain relief. Yoga, a form of gentle stretching, has also been found effective for pain relief. Viniyoga has been found to be superior to regular exercise for improving functional status and the use of pain medications. Pool therapy, in which the patients perform the physical therapy exercises in a swimming pool, can lessen the strain on sore muscles and help support the body while exercising.

Clinical Pearl	The use of cognitive behavioral therapy, progressive relaxation, exercise, interdisciplinary rehabilitation, functional restoration, and spinal manipulation have produced differences of 10 to 20 points on a 100-point visual analog scale.

Cognitive Behavioral Therapy

Many patients are interested in using the complementary methods of relaxation, biofeedback, self-hypnosis, and imagery to provide additional pain relief (APS, 2002; D'Arcy, 2007). Not all patients find these techniques to their liking. For those patients who are willing to invest the time and energy in learning how to use these methods, a good outcome can be expected. Music is an easy to use and greatly appreciated form of distraction and relaxation therapy. In early days music was incorporated into healing rituals. For pain relief music can be used in several different ways for example:

■ Using music as a part of physical therapy regimen can make the experience more pleasurable.
■ Music can be used to help structure breathing, provide a base for imagery, or provide another form of relaxation.
■ Playing or composing music can help express inner feelings and provide a creative outlet.

Even so simple an intervention as listening to pleasurable music can relax and help a patients feel pleasant memories. To achieve the best results with music therapy using music that the patient likes and prefers is best.

Relaxation

There are several different types of relaxation techniques that can be used to help control pain:

■ Regulating breathing, leading to decreased respiratory efforts
■ Relaxation tapes for progressive relaxation
■ Relaxation exercises (D'Arcy, 2007, 2010)

Relaxation techniques have been effective for decreasing pain (Cole & Brunk, 1999). These techniques result in the reduction of physical tension, muscle relaxation, and the promotion of emotional well-being (ASPMN, 2010; NCCAM, 2004). Using relaxation can be beneficial for patients who have chronic pain, cancer pain, and acute surgical pain (Dillard & Knapp, 2005). For patients who opt to use relaxation techniques some of the benefits include a heightened sense of well-being and improved scores on quality-of-life tools (Dillard & Knapp, 2005).

When patients use relaxation, they are asked to either progressively relax their muscles. Starting from the top of the body and progressing to the lower extremities, or focus on one process, such as controlling breathing. There are prerecorded tapes with relaxation exercises on them that patients can use at certain times of the day, such as when they feel stress building or as a help for relaxing to fall asleep. The patient can keep track of progress with a pain diary or journal.

Imagery

Imagery is a form of relaxation using a mental image. When a patient uses imagery, he or she is encouraged to create a peaceful or soothing image. The patient can enjoy the feeling of comfort that the scenario provides (ASPMN, 2010). Images can be created by the patient or provided by tapes if the patient has difficulty creating a useful mental image. As an example a patient could be asked to relax and picture a beautiful, ripe, tart lemon sitting on a counter in a sunny kitchen. The patient is asked to see the image, smell the fresh lemon scent, and taste the tartness of the fruit. This image is peaceful and pleasant. Patients should choose images that they can easily call up from memory so that they can use the technique very easily when it is needed for pain relief or stress reduction.

Using imagery for pain relief can also include the use of an image that locates the area of pain, such as with a headache. The patients can picture the headache as a red or dark color when pain is present. Working with the image, the patients can use relaxation and cognitive restructuring to see the headache lifting from the head, and getting smaller in size, or the color turning to a more peaceful and restful blue tone. This type of imagery is a little more complex, but patients can learn to use it effectively to help decrease pain.

The Arthritis Self-Management Program combines body-mind therapies, education and communication skills

- Education
- Cognitive restructuring
- Physical activity to reduce pain
- Problem solving
- Relaxation
- Development of communication skills to help interact with health care professionals (APS, 2002; D'Arcy, 2010)

The benefits of this program have demonstrated improved physical condition, long term pain reduction in a 4 year time period with a large cost savings that exceeds the initial cost of the program by 4 to 5 times. (Khatta, 2007) reduced pain that lasted over a 4-year time period and a cost savings of four to five times the cost of the program (Khatta, 2007).

Biofeedback, hypnosis, and meditation are other forms of relaxation techniques. Meditation, or mindfulness, has been found to reduce pain and help patients with chronic pain learn to cope more effectively with the condition (Khatta, 2007). If the patient can learn to quiet or center themselves to go through a series of images, or relaxation techniques, or focus on an object, meditation can be a useful adjunct for pain control. All of the mind–body techniques discussed previously have research support for their use, and which technique works for a specific patient depends on the type of approach the patient prefers.

Energy Therapy

Oriental cultures have used energy healing for many centuries. The idea of channeling energy from the universe through the patient to open blocked chakras is derived from the concept of Qigong, an external and internal energy life force. To use these therapies with patients in modern days, several newer energy therapies were developed to include Reiki, TT, and healing touch (Pierce, 2009).

There are some differences in the practices, but the overall concepts have a similar intent:

- The human body has an energy field that is generated from within the body to the outer world.
- There is a universal energy that flows through all living things, and it is available to them.
- Self-healing is promoted through the free flowing energy field.
- Disease and illness may be felt in the energy field and can be felt and changed by the healing intent of the practitioner (Pierce, 2009).

These energy therapies are effective for pain relief and relaxation. These therapies combine the best of the mind body holistic concept of CAM. Two of the most commonly practiced are Reiki and TT.

Reiki

The Reiki practitioner who is performing a therapeutic session on a patient uses the natural energy of the universe and channels through the patient's body to unblock chakras, or energy points. The techniques used by Reiki practitioners were developed and taught by the Buddhist monk Mikao Usui from Japan beginning in 1914 (Pierce, 2009). In basic Reiki, the Reiki practitioner places his or her hands in specific configurations on the patient's body to channel the universal energy through the chakras, opening up blocked points. In more advanced levels of practice, a Reiki practitioner transmits energy long distance to benefit a specific person (NCCAM, 2004).

Reiki has been used in Eastern cultures to ease both the mind and body. There are three levels of Reiki practice. Each level includes some additional form of energy transfer. Even with the basic level, the patient feels relaxed and experiences emotional and physical healing. The Reiki practitioner who channels the energy for the patient also receives some benefit: he or she may feel more relaxed and in tune with his or her own body energy after the session is completed.

Studies to determine the benefit of Reiki have focused on patients with cancer. In a study of 24 cancer patients using Reiki or rest periods, the Reiki patients had a significant decrease in pain (Pierce, 2009).

Therapeutic Touch

TT originated in the 1970s as a collaboration between two women: Dolores Krieger and Dora Kunz. The practice was based on concepts similar to Reiki. Although the two originators hoped that TT would become a part of standard patient care, it has proved more difficult to operationalize than anticipated (Pierce, 2009). At this time, the practice remains a nonstandard addition to patient care, though it is popular in some areas of the country.

TT is a form of energy medicine in which the practitioner does not touch the patient receiving the therapy, but rather focuses the energy on the patient's aura. Smoothing the aura by the energy transfer from the practitioner to the patient can help provide healing energy. It is often mistakenly referred to as "laying on of hands," which has a more religious connotation. The premise of TT is that the practitioner's healing force transfers or channels energy, thereby positively affecting the recovery of the patient (NCCAM, 2004). As the TT practitioner allows his or her hands to move over the patient, blocked energy is identified, and through the practitioner's hands, healing forces are directed to the area to promote healing and pain relief. There are five steps to TT:

- The practitioner takes time to relax and center their thoughts and mind
- Assessment, the next step is an overall assessment of the patient's external energy field
- The practitioner uses slow strokes down the patients energy field trying to unruffle and clear any energy blockage
- The fourth step concentrates energy into a specific area that is blocked
- The last step is an evaluation of the entire treatment process (Weintraub et al., 2008)

There are some studies that indicate greater pain relief with the use of TT in patients with chronic pain and fibromyalgia when compared with patient groups not receiving the energy treatment option (Pierce, 2009). It is difficult to conduct a study with TT because the recipient will know when they are not receiving the actual treatment but only a sham. Because randomized placebo-controlled studies are not possible with TT, it is difficult to measure the true effect of the practice. Currently more research is being done to help support the concept of energy therapy as a true source of relaxation, pain relief, and health promotion.

Nutritional Approaches

Folk medicine and natural healing have long been a part of most cultures. Herbal remedies are some of the most common forms of complementary therapeutics (Khatta, 2007). The advantage of these therapies is that they are simple and easy to use, are viewed as non-invasive, and are benign with few side effects; on the negative side, they have little or no quality control mechanism. Between the years of 1990 and 1997, herbal remedy use increased by 380% (Khatta, 2007). Costwise, the annual expenditure on herbal remedies in the United States exceeds 1.5 billion dollars (Khatta, 2007).

In early days the compounds were made by local entrepreneurs and sold door to door but today internet usage has made it easy to obtain just about any supplement or herbal remedy that a patient could want. The early compounds had no quality control. Many of these tonics and elixirs had cocaine or high alcohol contents, with flavorings to make them palatable. Laudanum was a popular elixir used for pain relief from childbirth to war injuries.

Today, all dietary supplements are categorized under the Dietary Supplement Health and Education Act of 1994, which requires quality, safety, and efficacy standards. However, there are still discrepancies in contents of some of the supplements and herbal remedies sold over the counter, so buyers should always be wary of what they are purchasing. This is especially true for pregnant and compromised patients. Common herbal remedies include:

- **Cayenne** (*Capsicum*). Capsaicin is the active ingredient of cayenne peppers (Khatta, 2007). Capsaicin, a cream made of the pepper extract, is sold as an over-the-counter cream, as a generic brand or with the brand name Zostrix at concentrations of 0.025% and 0.075%. The cream produces a strong sensation of heat, and it can also burn and sting. Patients who are using capsaicin should apply the cream three to four times daily over at least 2 weeks to see any improvement. When applying capsaicin cream, wearing gloves is advised and care with touching other parts of the body, especially the eyes, is recommended. A new 8% patch (Quetensa) is being marketed for treating intractable pain from PHN (See chapter 5 for more information). Capsaicin cream is recommended for use with:
  - Cluster headacahe
  - Psoriasis
  - Fibromyalgia
  - Pruritis
  - Itching and pain associated with postmastectomy pain syndrome
  - Postamputation pain
  - Neck pain (Weintraub et al., 2008)

- **Devil's claw** (*Harpagophytum procumbens*). Pain levels were reduced and functionality was increased in patients using this herb (Khatta, 2007).
- **Corydalis**. A frequently used herb, corydalis is an alkaloid with potent analgesic properties (Dillard & Knapp, 2005). It traditionally has been used for menstrual pain. Feverfew is being used for migraine prophyaxis. In a review of 5 placebo controlled studies feverfew was found to be superior to placebo (Weintraub et al., 2008).

Nutritional Supplements

- One of the most popular and disputed supplements for arthritis pain is glucosamine and chondroitin. Studies have shown a slowing of disease progression over time and that combination medications can affect pain in osteoarthritis patients (Khatta, 2007).
- Omega-3 fatty acids affect prostaglandin metabolism, thereby affecting the inflammatory process. Fish oil has been found to have anti-inflammatory effects in patients with rheumatoid arthritis, whereas flaxseed oil has not had similar effect (Khatta, 2007). Alpha-Lipoic acid was found to be useful and reduce symptom scores for patients with peripheral neuropathies and diabetic neuropathy (Weintraub et al., 2008)
- The use of iron supplements has produced positive results in patients with restless leg syndrome because low ferritin levels were found to be correlated with higher symptom burden and decreased symptoms after iron repletion. Caution with iron supplements is advised to avoid iron overload as it has been associated with increased cancer and other debilitating chronic conditions (Weintraub et al., 2008).

Clinical Pearl   Patients who are taking nutritional supplements and herbal remedies should tell their primary care provider that they are using the substances. Because there is the potential for drug–drug interactions with mainstream medications, every patient should be asked if they are taking a supplement or herbal remedy. Only those supplements and herbs that have shown efficacy in clinical trials and are recommended by the NCCAM should be used for complementary pain relief.

SUMMARY

CAM therapies can be very helpful in decreasing pain, relieving stress and enhancing relaxation. Music, storytelling, humor, massage, yoga and distraction are among a few of additional techniques. Most are benign and can only offer positive support for the medical regimen. Each patient is an individual and because there are many to choose from, every patient should be able to find a good CAM therapy to complement his or her conventional therapy.

Case Study

Jeff Smith, age 46, fell from a ladder at work and hurt his back. He has had back surgery to repair the damage from the fall, but he still continues to have pain. He has been diagnosed with failed back syndrome, and he has not been able to get back to work. He is currently taking extended release opioid medications—MS-Contin, 45 mg twice per day—with a short-acting medication, Vicodin, for breakthrough pain. He also takes a muscle relaxant and an antidepressant. He complains that the medications are making him feel sleepy and fuzzy headed all the time. He sleeps during the day when he takes his medication and cannot sleep at night because of the pain that increases when he stays in bed for longer than a few hours.

His primary care provider sends Jeff to you to see if there are any other ways to treat his pain and to get an opinion about continuing to prescribe the opioids. When you speak to Jeff he tells you, "I hate those pills, but they're the only thing that helps me get through the day. I always have pain, but when I take the medication, it helps dull the pain sensation. I'm awake all night watching television. I can't stand to lie in bed. I sleep in a chair. I feel like my back is tight, and it really starts to ache. My whole life is turning upside down. I would like to retrain for a job where I wouldn't have to do so much physical work, but I can't because I sleep all day. Do you have any suggestions for helping me with this pain?"

1. Considering the type of medications that the patient is on, should there be an adjustment of his medications? Are the medications producing the expected outcome? Will you consider decreasing the medication doses with CAM?
2. What CAM techniques would be helpful for Jeff?
3. When you mention physical therapy to Jeff, he balks and says, "I have been there before, and it just hurts too bad to do the exercises." What types of adjustment could you make for Jeff or what different types of physical therapy could you offer Jeff?
4. As Jeff progresses with his CAM therapies, he feels he can decrease his medications. How would you taper Jeff's medications and still maintain adequate pain control?
5. What are the benefits of offering Jeff CAM therapies in addition to his regular medication management?

REFERENCES

American Pain Society. (2002). *Guideline for the management of pain in osteoarthritis, rheumatoid arthritis, and juvenile chronic arthritis.* Glenview, IL: American Pain Society.

American Pain Society. (2005). *Guideline for the management of fibromyalgia pain syndrome in adults and children.* Glenview, IL: American Pain Society.

American Pain Society. (2006). *Pain control in the primary care setting.* Glenview, IL: American Pain Society.

American Society of Pain Management Nurses. (2010). *Core curriculum for pain management nursing.* Philadelphia, PA: WB Saunders.

Berry, P., Covington, E., Dahl, J., Katz, J., & Miaskowski, C. (2006). *Pain: Current understanding of assessment, management, and treatments.* Reston, VA: National Pharmaceutical Council, Inc.

Bruckenthal, P., & D'Arcy, Y. (2007). A complementary approach to pain management. *Topics in Advanced Practice Nursing eJournal, 7*(1). Retrieved from http://www.medscape.com/viewarticle/556408

Cole, B. H., & Brunk, Q. (1999). Holistic interventions for acute pain episodes: An integrative review. *Journal of Holistic Nursing, 17*(4), 384–396.

D'Arcy, Y. (2007). *Pain management: Evidence-based tools and techniques for nursing professionals.* Marblehead, MA: HCPro.

Dillard, J., & Knapp, S. (2005). Complementary and alternative pain therapy in the emergency department. *Emergency Medical Clinics of North America, 23,* 529–549.

French, S. D., Cameron, M., Walker, B. F., Reggars, J. W., & Esterman, A. J. (2006). Superficial heat or cold for low-back pain. *Cochrane Database for Systemic Reviews,* (2), 2006.

Furlan, A. D., Brosseau, L., Imamura, M., & Irvin E. (2002). Massage for low-back pain. *Cochrane Database for Systematic Reviews,* (2), 2006.

Khatta, M. (2007). A complementary approach to pain management. *Topics in Advanced Practice Nursing eJournal, 7*(1). Retrieved from http://www.medscape.com/viewarticle/556408

National Center for Complementary and Alternative Medicine. (2004). *Expanding horizons of health care strategic plan 2005–2009.* Bethesda, MD: U.S. Department of Health and Human Services. National Institutes of Health. Retrieved from www.nccam.nih.gov

Pierce, B. (2009). A nonpharmacologic adjunct for pain management. *The Nurse Practitioner, 34*(2), 10–13.

Weintraub, M., Mamtani, R., & Micozzi, M. (2008). *Complementary and integrative medicine in pain management.* New York, NY: Springer Publishing Company.

7

Pain Clinic Referrals and Interventional Options

OVERVIEW

There are various interventional options for pain relief that are performed by pain specialists who are affiliated with pain clinics. When looking at which type of intervention is best (e.g., injection, rehabilitation), it is important to assess what type of pain the patient is experiencing to determine which clinic to recommend for the intervention option that would be best for the patient. For example, if the patient has a radicular pain that is the result of spinal nerve impingement, an epidural steroid injection might be recommended. A referral for consultation to an injection clinic or specialist would be appropriate in this case. If the patient has nonradicular low back pain, a referral to a rehabilitation or physical medicine and rehabilitation clinic might be recommended. The goal in this case is to maximize the patient's functionality.

SELECTING A PAIN CLINIC

The type of clinic selected is highly dependent on the type of practitioners who work in the clinic. Some examples of clinics that are especially designed to treat pain include the following:

- *Anesthesia-based clinics*, where anesthesiologists provide various interventional pain management options, such as epidural steroid injections

■ *Interdisciplinary or multidisciplinary clinics*, which are made up of anesthesiologists, physiatrists, rehabilitation specialists, nurses, physical therapists, psychologists, and so forth, and where the patient receives specialized therapy, depending on the pain condition

■ *Rehabilitation clinics*, where the clinic staff are trained to help patients manage their pain and return to work, focusing on mobility and reconditioning

■ *Specialty clinics*, which are focused on a specific type of pain, such as headache (International Association for the Study of Pain [IASP], 2008)

Since 1950, when the first pain clinic was started, chronic pain patients have benefited from having access to a specialist who is interested in treating chronic pain conditions. As these clinics became popular with both patients and referring physicians, the number of pain clinics grew dramatically to 1,200 pain facilities in 1987, and even more dramatically from 2,650 to 3,000 pain facilities today.

Considering the large number of patients with chronic low back pain alone, the number of clinics still is insufficient to meet the increasing demand for services. Most chronic pain conditions are treated at the onset in primary care practices. The health care provider tries to bring the pain under control with medications, physical therapy, and other treatment options that are known to be useful for the condition. For most patients, this approach will work, but only 58% of patients with chronic pain are satisfied with their analgesics (American Pain Foundation, 2005). For many patients with chronic pain, an interventional option with or without medication management may be needed to help relieve or decrease pain and increase functionality.

GUIDELINES FOR PAIN CLINIC REFERRAL

In general, a pain clinic referral is indicated when the following occurs:

■ The patient has had a number of medications that have failed to relieve the pain, even though doses have been adjusted and other medications have been tried.

■ The patient continues to complain of severe level pain and cannot comply with the expected treatment regimen, such as physical therapy sessions.

■ The health care provider is unsure about continuing a treatment regimen or needs confirmation that a certain treatment regimen is the correct approach to treating the patient's pain.

■ The patient seems to have a condition that persists, such as radicular back pain, and may be helped by an interventional pain management technique, such as an epidural steroid injection. Many primary care practitioners feel that once they have reached the end of their medication options a referral for a pain clinic evaluation may be helpful to determine if there are other pain management options for the patient. The evaluation can also lend support to the current plan of care and diagnosis.

When considering a referral to a pain clinic, these criteria are helpful to use to ensure that the clinic will provide the services that the patient needs (see Exhibit 7.1 for desirable characteristics of a pain clinic). It is helpful to remember that the success of the clinic referral relies on the communication between the health care professional making the referral for treatment or evaluation and the pain

---

Exhibit 7.1

Desirable Characteristics of a Pain Clinic

A pain clinic should have the following characteristics:

■ Access/regular interaction with at least three types of medical specialties or health care providers, including a psychiatrist or psychologist
■ Regular, patient-related communication
■ Both diagnostic and therapeutic services
■ Records maintained so that patient outcomes can be tracked
■ Practitioners knowledgeable in basic sciences and clinical practices related to pain management
■ Patient referrals and emergencies handled by a trained health care professional
■ Providers licensed in the country and state in which they practice

Source: Adapted from International Association for the Study of Pain, 2008.

specialist. Each provider should communicate any changes in the patient's treatment regimen, such as medication changes, any procedures that are performed, and any new information that is found during assessment or treatment.

No matter what the size or specialty of the clinic, the patient with chronic pain will benefit from the thorough assessment and evaluation process that is part of the specialist visit. When an interventional option is chosen to help relieve pain, the choice is made after a multidimensional assessment and evaluation process that is designed to help pinpoint options that will best help relieve the patient's pain and assist the patient in coping with the chronic pain.

There are a wide variety of interventional methods for pain relief that include the following:

- Epidural steroid injections and facet joint injections
- Prolotherapy
- Radio frequency lesioning
- Intradiscal electrotherapy (IDET)
- Epiduroscopy
- Spinal cord stimulators
- Implanted intrathecal pumps

Depending on the pain complaint and the condition of the patient, the pain specialist will select an option that will provide the biggest benefit to the patient. More information on specific interventions will be provided in the following sections of the chapter.

Evaluation by a Pain Specialist for Interventional Pain Management

All patients who are seen for evaluation in a pain clinic or by a pain specialist undergo a panel of tests and assessments that are designed to help determine the best approach to the pain problem. Patients with chronic pain have been seen by any number of surgeons, psychiatrists, physical therapists, and primary care physicians. They are usually very familiar with pain medications, the type of pain they are experiencing, and what will make the pain better or worse.

A detailed medical history will also be taken that may include some or all of these components:

- Past pain experiences
- Current or past chemical use, illicit or prescription substance abuse, or a history of a substance abuse disorder
- Medical history
- Surgical history
- Psychiatric history
- Medication use history
- Laboratory findings
- Imaging results (e.g., computed tomography [CT] scans or magnetic resonance imaging [MRI])
- Other pertinent workup results (e.g., electromyography)

Because most of these patients will have been through many examinations, they may feel this is one more time when they will be told that there is little that can be done. Encouraging the patient to be very open to the experience will help set a positive tone for the patient's visit. Taking the time to listen to the patient describe their pain and what has worked and what has not been beneficial will pay a large dividend. Establishing a positive relationship with the patient and the referring practitioner from the beginning of the process will help ensure that the best outcomes will be achieved at the end of the treatment period.

INJECTIONS AS PAIN INTERVENTION

Spinal Injections (Figure 7.1)

There are various reasons that spinal injection therapy can provide pain relief for patients:

- Age-related changes in the spine can create bone spurs and facet arthropathy that can result in nerve impingement or degenerative disc disease where, as the disc dries out, the associated nerve can be compressed by the vertebral body.
- Some patients who have back surgery do not get the expected result of pain relief. These patients are said to have "failed back syndrome." Injections can help relieve the pain of the nerve damage

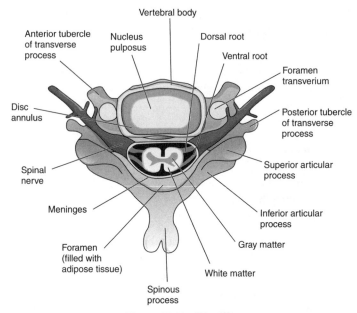

Figure 7.1 ■ Vertebra

or impingement. Additional surgery may not provide any additional benefit at this point so reducing the pain to a tolerable level would be a reasonable goal.

■ Back injury that causes a tear in the annulus surrounding the disc resulting in a herniated disc or HNP the herniated material presses on the adjacent nerve root causing pain; this is commonly called *sciatica*.

■ Conditions such as spinal stenosis caused by age related changes to the spinal bones thickening the vertebral walls and narrowing the spinal canal. These changes cause deep midback pain with radicular pain down one or both legs causing a gait disturbance, pain, and decreased mobility.

Some injections are performed as a treatment, whereas others may be used as a diagnostic tool. Because injections are an elective option, a risk/benefit analysis is done to ensure the benefit does outweigh the risk and that the patient fully understands potential outcomes. There are certain conditions that preclude the use of injections, such as infection or anticoagulation (Wallace & Staats, 2005). The final step before the procedure is performed is providing a risk benefit analysis to the patient and obtaining informed consent from the patient.

Epidural Steroid Injections

Steroid injections can be performed at almost any level of the spine. Most commonly, they are done under fluoroscopy to properly locate the nerve that is being affected and to target the injection site. The solution used for the injection combines preservative free medications; a local anesthetic such as bupivacine or ropivacaine and a steroid. Using this provides immediate and localized relief if successful. The local anesthetic works first while the steroid can take up to week to provide pain relief. Since the medication is injected directly onto the nerve root the pain relief is targeted to the nerve root causing the pain.

Most patients need to have the injection preauthorized by their insurance provider to ensure coverage. A series of three to six injections (the annual number for most pain specialists) is commonly performed. The first injection may decrease the pain or there may be partial relief that subsequent injections may improve.

To perform an epidural steroid injection, the anesthesia pain specialist will position the patient to allow access to the affected area, usually in a sitting position with the back arched. Once the sterile field is ready and the injection area has been prepared and treated with local anesthetic, the injection is performed into the epidural space of the nerve or into the facet joint that is producing the pain (Figure 7.2). The ASIPP systematic review report the evidence for various types of blocks to be:

■ Caudal blocks-strong evidence for short term pain relief and moderate for long term relief. Evidence for efficacy in spinal stenosis is not strong

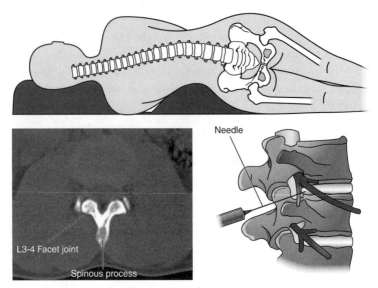

Figure 7.2 ■ Facet injection

- Interlaminar blocks for lumbar radiculopathy—strong short term evidence with limited long term relief
- Selective nerve root injections moderate relief
- Facet joint injections—medial branch blocks—moderate evidence for short term and long term improvement (Trescott, 2009)

Trigger/Tender Point Injections

When a patient can point to a specific spot that is painful a trigger or tender point injection can be used to decrease pain in the area. There is some indication of efficacy in myofascial syndromes. To perform the procedure, local anesthetic (lidocaine) is injected directly into the painful area. Because injection of tender points in fibromyalgia is not supported by research, several national guidelines, such as the American Pain Society Fibromyalgia Pain Guidelines, do not recommend tender point injection for fibromyalgia patients but clinically they are used for pain relief at tender points.

Botulinum Toxin (Botox) Injections

Botulinum toxins are produced by the anaerobic bacteria *Clostridium botulinum*. There are several different types of neurotoxins (Botox, Myobloc) that can be used for the U.S. Food and Drug Administration (FDA)-approved purpose of treating the pain of cervical dystonia.

To use a Botox injection to treat cervical dystonia pain, the toxin is injected directly into a muscle, with muscle weakness occurring within 2 weeks. There is a gradual resolution of the weakness with a slow return to normal. The clinical effect is reported to be at most 3 months. Pain relief from an injection is reported as greater than the neuromuscular blocking effect. The recommended treatment interval is 12 weeks.

Other conditions that are not FDA approved in which anecdotal reports indicate that Botox has been used effectively include the following:

- Relief of migraine headaches was discovered as a side effect of the use of Botox for plastic surgery injections. In a study of plastic surgery patients who received Botox for cosmetic purposes, 51% of 77 patients with migraine reported complete relief of headache and 38% of 77 patients reported partial relief. Other headache types where Botox has been used include tension, cluster, and chronic daily headaches.
- Relief of musculoskeletal pain, including chronic temporomandibular joint dysfunction, chronic cervicothoracic pain, chronic low back pain, and pyriformis syndrome.

OTHER THERAPIES

Less commonly, a procedure that affects nerve roots, such as radiofrequency lesioning or IDET, or one that affects specific muscle groups, such as prolotherapy, may be used. There is limited research available for these techniques, and support may not be strong as a result. This does not mean these techniques have no value, but that the research literature support may be sparse. For most of these techniques, the intervention is placed directly at the source or site of the pain. These are not first-line therapies and are just options that some pain specialists have found to be helpful for pain relief.

Radiofrequency Lesioning

This therapy uses a heated probe to deliver radiofrequency thermal energy to the painful disc. The process compresses and coagulates disc material and has been found to be most useful for patients who have an internally disrupted disc (Raj, 2008).

To perform the procedure, a cannula is inserted into the intervertebral disc. A catheter is inserted through the cannula and passed into the outer disc tissue. Current is then passed through the electrode, heating the surrounding tissue and eliminating the source of the pain (Raj, 2008).

Intradiscal Electrothermal Therapy

To perform IDET, the patient receives conscious sedation. From the nonpainful side, a 17-gauge needle is inserted into the disc through the annulus to the site of the pain. A catheter is then threaded through the needle and the catheter tip is heated to 90°F over the span of 13 minutes (Raj, 2008). The process reduces the size of annular fissures, increases the stability of the disc, and destroys nociceptors in the annular walls, stopping nociceptive input of pain stimuli (Raj, 2008). This is an outpatient procedure; the patient should be able to return home when recovered from sedation.

This practice has provided anecdotal reports of pain relief for discogenic back pain. In a randomized, double blind, controlled trial of IDET versus placebo, the study outcomes demonstrated no significant benefit for the IDET patients over the placebo group (Freeman et al., 2005). This type of therapy should not be used as a first-line option, but reserved for use when other pain management options have failed to provide adequate pain relief.

Both radiofrequency lesioning and IDET have associated risks and benefits. The patient must be informed that even though pain relief is the goal, there is a risk of nerve root injuries, catheter breakage, disc herniation, infection, epidural abscess, and spinal cord damage (Raj, 2008).

Prolotherapy or Regenerative Injection Therapy

Prolotherapy is classed as a regenerative therapy aimed at creating an inflammatory response that will raise growth factor levels promoting tissue repair or growth. The injection of an hypertonic dextrose solution or an irritant solution, such as dextrose/phenol/glycerine or pumice, into weakened back muscles to promote tissue repair and correct tendon and muscle laxity has been found to be an effective means of pain relief when combined with an aggressive physical therapy regimen. Additionally this type of therapy can be used as a joint injection or for soft tissue healing. In a study of low back pain patients who were treated with prolotherapy, 3 months after treatment there was a 60% increase in collagen fibril diameter, decreased pain, and increased range of motion (Weintraub, Mamtani, Micozzi, 2008).

There are several conditions for which this technique has been implemented, including:

- Discogenic back pain
- Chronic pain from ligament or tendons resulting from repetitive motion disorder
- Osteoarthritis
- Cervical, thoracic, lumbar, lumbosacral, and sacroiliac instability the use of anti-inflammatory medication such as NSAIDs is discouraged to control the pain of the injections since the purpose of the injection is to create a low grade inflammatory process

Epiduroscopy

Epiduroscopy involves the insertion of a fiber optic scope into the epidural space of the spine. It is used as a last line for treating low back pain. On the scope inserted into the epidural space scope are tools that can be used to remove scar tissue from nerve roots. Overall, the epidural adhesiolysis technique has only limited success. The evidence for using spinal endoscopy is strong for short term relief and moderate for long term improvement of refractory low back pain (Trescot, 2009).

Implanted Modalities
Implanted Intrathecal Pumps

When a patient gets to the point that medications and interventions such as epidural steroid injections are not working to control pain and functionality is heavily impaired a pain specialist may consider implanting an intrathecal pump. These pumps an be used for chronic pain or oncology pain management. The guide for pump placement in oncology patients is a survival expectancy of greater than 3 months (Figure 7.3). This technique is not a first-line option. There should be considerable trial use of other techniques for pain management before consideration of an implanted pump.

The technique consists of an implanted computerized pump that can be set by the pain specialist to deliver. The medication is placed

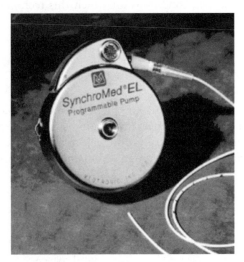

Figure 7.3 ■ Intrathecal pump. *Source:* Used with permission of Medtronic, Inc.

into a reservoir in the pump. The computer chip in the pump has the settings that are entered by the pain specialist that tells the pumps how to deliver the medication. It can be programmed to deliver a continuous rate most commonly but the pumps have the option of reducing or increasing flow rates at certain times of the day if programmed for variable flow. Medication flows from the pump to the intrathecal space by a flexible catheter that is tunneled from the spinal insertion point along the lateral aspect of the patient's body and connected to the pump. The pump is placed into a pocket usually on the patient's abdomen below the belt line or other subcutaneous tissue close to the skin's surface to facilitate refilling the pump.

Pump refills are done when needed, according to the concentration and the infusion rate of the medication. A refill kit with a specialized needle is used to withdraw any leftover medication from the pump reservoir, and new medication is inserted into the pump reservoir. The pump refill date is then reset to a new date that is set using the information on the concentration and delivery rate.

Medications that are FDA-approved for use in implanted intrathecal pumps are as follows:

- Morphine
- Baclofen (Lioresal)
- Ziconotide (Prialt)

All medications used in implanted intrathecal pumps should be free of preservative. Morphine is the most common medication, and using an intrathecal medication delivery can provide morphine doses that are 300 times as potent as oral morphine (D'Arcy, 2010; Wallace & Staats, 2005). In order to test the feasibility of using an implanted pump there should be a trial with an external catheter places either intrathecally or epidurally to assure that there will be benefit for the patients. During the trial period, the drug selection is based on the following:

- History of opioid tolerance
- Side effect history
- Pain afferent spinal cord level compared with catheter tip location (Wallace & Staats, 2005)

The lipophilicity of the selected pain medication, the available lipid supply of the spinal cord, and the accessibility of the cerebrospinal fluid and blood supply can directly affect the analgesic action of the medication being used (D'Arcy, 2010; Wallace & Staats, 2005). Ziconotide (Prialt) is a unique medication classed as a neuronal-type calcium channel blocker. For medical use the venom of the marine cone snail is used as an continuous intrathecal infusion (Lynch, Cheng, & Yee, 2006). It can be effective for chronic and neuropthic pain conditions (Schroeder et al., 2006). There are some specific side effects, mainly neuropsychiatric, that can be significant. These include the following:

- Depression
- Cognitive impairment
- Depressed levels of consciousness
- Hallucinations
- Elevated creatinine kinase levels (Lynch, Cheng, & Yee, 2006)

Prialt use should be reserved for patients who have failed all other more conventional medications and interventions.

Practitioners run the risk of pump malfunction if other medications than the approved three are used in the pump (see Exhibit 7.2 for guidelines in selecting a candidate for intrathecal medication delivery).

Intrathecal medication use should be carefully considered before the pump is implanted. In a study of 202 patients with refractory cancer pain the decrease was determined to be 20% after pump implantation measured by pain ratings on a VAAS scale (de Leon-Casasola, 2009). A side benefit of IT therapy in this study was a reduction in constipation and impaired consciousness. As a rule of thumb if the patient does not have at least a 50% pain severity reduction while the pump trial is taking place, placing the device should be reconsidered. The patient risk–benefit ratio should be carefully weighed, and all other reasonable options should be tried before the pump implantation is tried. If the patient does not have a 50% reduction in pain levels with the prepump implantation trial, the final implantation should be reconsidered. There are

| |
| |

Exhibit 7.2

Criteria for Selecting a Candidate for Intrathecal Medication Delivery

In general, the successful candidate for referral for implanted intrathecal pump and intrathecal medication delivery includes the patient for whom:

- Oral analgesia with multiple oral or transcutaneous trials, including dose titration, has been ineffective
- Side effects, despite opioid rotation, are intolerable
- Functional analgesia took effect and provided benefit during temporary trial infusion
- Psychological stability and reasonable goals can be demonstrated
- Access to care is manageable: the patient is to return to the pain clinic for pump refills and dose adjustments
- Acceptance of the procedure has been demonstrated
- Intractable spasticity was unrelieved by oral antispasmodics and spasticity was improved with baclofen test dosing

Source: Adapted from Wallace & Staats, 2005, p. 342.

---

some risks that the patient should be aware of before the catheter is placed (see Exhibit 7.3 for risks related to intrathecal medication administration).

Spinal Cord Stimulation

Neurostimulation for the relief of pain was noted as early as 2,500 BC in Egypt where electric catfish or torpedo fish with electric shocking capacity of 220 volts were placed on painful areas hoping to relieve pain (Junkin, Lynch, Beradoni, 2009). The concept of spinal cord stimulation is based on the idea that using a non-noxious stimulus can reduce pain perception (Lynch et al., 2009) It is also thought that the sympathetic nervous system is activated by the pulse generation of the stimulator and that additional neuronal

Exhibit 7.3

Risks and Considerations when Evaluating the Candidacy of a Patient for Intrathecal Medication Administration

Risks and considerations for patient candidacy include the following:

- Does the patient have any placement issues, such as spinal deformity, past spinal surgery, or abdominal surgery, that would make placement difficult?
- All patients are at risk for infection, meningitis, arachnoiditis, and catheter-related granuloma formation.
- Anticoagulation can cause a compressive hematoma when the catheter is being placed or removed.
- Pump malfunction can cause a withdrawal syndrome.
- Low pressure spinal headaches may occur.
- There may be a need for dose escalation and the development of tolerance.

Source: Adapted from Wallace & Staats, 2005; D'Arcy, 2010.

pathways may be activated and provide additional pain relief (Wallace & Staats, 2005).

Most spinal cord stimulators use a low volt battery, similar to a pacemaker battery, connected to two or more leads that are implanted into the epidural space in the area determined to be the pain generator. These leads are placed either percutaneously or laminectomy. When activated the patient will experience a mild tingling sensation in the painful area. Many patients feel that this sensation is similar to a transcutaneous electrical nerve stimulator (TENS) unit. (Mailis-Gagnon et al., 2008; Figure 7.4).

Conditions that have found SCS to be helpful for pain relief include:

- Peripheral vascular disease
- Refractory angina
- Chronic pancreatitis

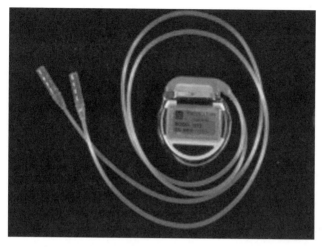

Figure 7.4 ■ SPS pulse generator. *Source:* Used with permission of Medtronic, Inc.

- Chronic pelvic pain
- Facial pain
- Idiopathic foot pain
- Failed back syndrome
- Chronic neuropathic pain; complex regional pain syndrome, phantom limb pain, diabetic neuropathy, radiculitis, post-thoracotomy pain postherpetic neuralgia (Mailis-Gagnon et al., 2008; McJunkin et al., 2009; Neuromodulation Therapy Access Coalition [NTAC], 2008).

Patients who are being considered for SCS should be given a very thorough physical and psychological examination. They should have used medication management and trialed combinations and doses of medication with limited results. Although the research results are not strong it is covered by Medicare, other government health care programs, all major commercial health plans, and most worker's compensation plans in the United States (D'Arcy, 2010). The chance that SCS will work and increase function is an outcome that should be considered if the trial stimulation relieves pain. The last positive

Table 7.1 ■ *Criteria for Appropriate Patient Selection for SCS*

Indications for Appropriate Patient Selection	Conditions Contraindicating Patient Selection
■ Persistent pain despite exhaustion of all acceptable and less invasive treatment options ■ Patient psychiatric evaluation has ruled out psychiatric comorbidities, issues of substance abuse, and potential for secondary gain ■ Diagnosis has been established for the pain ■ Test stimulation trial indicates a good level of pain relief and functional improvement	■ Coagulopathy ■ Sepsis ■ Untreated major comorbidity, such as depression ■ Serious drug or behavior problem ■ Inability to cooperate or control the device ■ Potential for secondary gain ■ "Demand" cardiac pacemaker in place ■ Comorbid condition requiring possible future MRI. Pregnant or lactating women

Source: Adapted from McJunkin et al., 2009; NTAC, 2008; Wallace & Staats, 2005.

aspect of SCS is that it is minimally invasive, reversible, and nondestructive, and if the neuromodulation does not provide the expected result, the lead(s) and generator can be explanted (D'Arcy, 2010; NTAC, 2008) (Table 7.1).

With both implanted techniques, patient selection and preimplantation medication manipulation and dose adjustment should all be tried prior to considering an implanted modality. Because the device mat require frequent adjustment the patient needs to commit to follow-up visits. Choosing the right technique and the right patient will provide more positive outcomes.

Returning the Patient to the Referring Practice

When the patient returns to the referring practice after treatment by a pain clinic, it is essential to let the patient know you are comfortable with the treatment regimen that the pain clinic specialist has prescribed. By presenting a united front to the patient, there is little room for any deviation from the plan, unless the practitioners and patient agree to an adjustment.

Establishing good communication with the pain clinic specialists will be especially important once the patient is no longer being seen in their clinic. If the practitioner who refers the patient has a good understanding of the medication or therapy regimen, there is no reason that the primary care provider cannot provide the same level of pain management care. It is also important for the two practitioners to have access to current records to confirm medications, dosages, and any adjustments that were made to the plan of care.

Mabel Jones is a 57-year-old patient who was in a car accident 2 years ago and had significant trauma to her back and chest. She has had multiple back surgeries, and at the time of the accident, a thoracotomy was performed. She has been seeing her surgeon and her primary care health care provider for several years, and they have been managing her pain with short-acting opioids, such as oxycodone and hydrocodone with acetaminophen. She is still complaining of significant pain in her back and down her legs, and she has some areas on her chest wall that have what she describes as a burning sensation. Her health care provider has manipulated her medications many times, tried several different types and classes of medications, and now feels that Mabel would benefit from a pain clinic referral to make sure they are doing all that they can do to help alleviate the pain.

When Mabel sees the pain specialist, she asks Mabel to fill out a multidimensional pain assessment form, talks to her about her medications and how they work, and does a complete examination and reviews the most current x-rays, MRIs, and CT results. When she speaks to Mabel about her pain, Mabel tells the pain specialist, "The pain is always there. It really never goes away. If I have to stand or walk any distance, I really feel the pain down my legs. On most days, I can live with the pain at about a 5/10, but when it gets higher than that, I really have a hard time. When it gets like that, the pain medicine doesn't work too well. It takes so long to work. Then I have this nagging burning pain in my chest since I had the accident and surgery. It feels like someone is holding a match to my chest right in that spot. It really bothers me, and I can't sleep too well because of it. I wish I had never gone out to shop on that day. If only I had not had that accident, I might have an entirely different life now."

Mabel's current medications are as follows:
- oxycodone with acetaminophen: two tablets 3 times per day
- zolpidem for sleep
- ibuprofen for her back pain as needed

Questions to Consider

1. What type of pain does Mabel have? More than one type? How do you know there are different types of pain? Will the type of pain she has make a difference in how the pain specialist treats her pain?
2. Will changing her medications to a long-acting opioid medication with a short-acting medication benefit Mabel? Should there be other types of medications that are used for her pain?
3. What types of interventional options would be helpful for Mabel?
4. Because of the mixed nature of Mabel's pain, what is the best way to treat each component?
5. Does Mabel have any contraindications for use of interventional options for pain relief?

REFERENCES

American Pain Foundation. (2005). *Pain facts: An overview of American pain surveys.*

de Leon-Casasola, O. & Rauck, R. (2009). Intrathecal therapy for the management of cancer and noncancer pain. *Pain Medicine News, 7*(12):75–78.

Freeman, B. J., Fraser, R. D., Cain, C. M., Hall, D. J., & Chappie, D. C. (2005). A randomized, double blind, controlled trial: Intradiscal electrothermal therapy versus placebo for the treatment of chronic discogenic low back pain. *Spine, 30*(21), 2369–2377.

International Association for the Study of Pain. (2008). Retrieved from www.iasp.org

Lynch, S. S., Cheng, C. M., & Yee, J. L. (2006). Intrathecal ziconotide for refractory chronic pain. *Annals of Pharmacotherapy, 40*(7–8), 1293–1300.

Mailis-Gagnon, A., Furlan, A., Sandoval, J. A., & Taylor, R. (2008). Spinal cord stimulation for chronic pain. *The Cochrane Database of Systemic Reviews, 3.*

McJunkin, T., Lynch, P., & Berardoni N. (2009). Neurostimulation for pain. *Pain Medicine News, 7*(12):9–14.

Neuromodulation Therapy Access Coalition (NTAC). (2008). *Position statement on spinal cord neuromodulation.* Retrieved from www.aapm.org

Raj, P. P. (2008). Intervertebral disc: Anatomy-physiology-pathophysiology-treatment. *Pain Practice, 8*(1), 18–44.

Schroeder, C. I., Doering, C. J., Zamponi, G. W., & Lewis, R. J. (2006). N-type calcium channel blockers: Novel therapeutics for the treatment of pain. *Medicinal Chemistry, 2*(5), 535–543.

Trescott, A. (2009, December). Interventional approaches to the management of spinal pain. *Pain Medicine News,* pp. 85–95.

Wallace, M., & Staats, P. (2005). *Pain medicine and management.* New York, NY: McGraw-Hill.

Weintraub, M., Mamtani, R., & Micozzi, M. (2008). *Complementary and integrative medicine in pain management.* New York, NY: Springer Publishing Company.

ADDITIONAL RESOURCES

Abram, S. E., & O'Connor, T. C. (1996). Complications associated with epidural steroid injections. *Regional Anesthesia, 21*(2), 149–162.

Armon, C., Argoff, C. E., Samuels, J., & Backonja, M. M. (2007). Assessment: Use of epidural steroid injections to treat radicular lumbosacral pain: Report of the therapeutics and technology assessment subcommittee of the American Academy of Neurology. *Neurology, 68*(10), 723–729.

DePalma, M. J., Bhargava, A., & Slipman, C. W. (2008). A critical appraisal of the evidence for selective nerve root injection in the treatment of lumbosacral radiculopathy. *Archives of Physical Medicine and Rehabilitation, 86*(7), 1477–1483.

McCarberg, B. H., Nicholson, B. D., Todd, K. H., Palmer, T., & Penles, L. (2007). The impact of pain on quality of life and the unmet needs of pain management: Results from pain sufferers and physicians participating in an internet survey. *American Journal of Therapeutics, 15*(4), 312–320.

III

Special Considerations for Treating Chronic Pains

8

Effect of Opioid Polymorphisms and Gender Differences

OVERVIEW

One of the newest pieces of pain management research is focused on the effect of the patient's gender and genetic makeup on pain medication binding and utilization. For many years, there has been speculation by clinicians as to why some patients responded well to small doses of opioids and got excellent pain relief, whereas other patients required large doses to get even minimal pain relief.

For many years, a patient was considered drug seeking if large doses of medication were required to control pain. Patients were considered to be exemplary if they could manage pain relief with small amounts of medication. Little concern was given to the individual differences that all patients bring to the pain management setting. Because little was known about how genetics, sex, gender, and pain were related, the patient often felt that he/she was being blamed for any lack of success with pain management regimens.

Today, we know that pain relief is not a single entity based on putting the right medication into the right patient, but one more reliant on patient genetics and pathophysiology. As noted in Chapter 4, not all patients can utilize certain pain medications, such as codeine, because they lack the liver enzyme needed to convert the medication to morphine, the active form. As research progresses, findings indicate that there are many genetic factors that play an important role in how pain medications work for the individual patient.

Patients with chronic pain also have a changed response to subsequent pain stimulus because the repeated pain stimuli cause the nervous system to modify its function to react more comprehensively. This is called *neuronal plasticity* (Rowbotham, Kidd, & Porreca, 2006). Neuronal plasticity can result in the phenomenon called *peripheral sensitization*, in which nociception in peripheral neurons is heightened and pain stimuli are felt to be more severe than is indicated by the stimulus. As the pain input continues, pain-facilitating substances such as cytokines and substance P are recruited to the area, leading to increased pain sensation, inflammation, and the development of hyperalgesia and allodynia.

Wind-up is another physiologic change that occurs when the central nervous system pain response is activated because of continued peripheral pain input. As the pain continues, the wind-up phenomenon allows the patient to experience pain that is more intense, prolonged, and much more difficult to treat. With wind-up, the *N*-methyl d-aspartate (NMDA) receptors are activated and help accelerate and increase the intensity of the pain stimuli. Examples of diseases where wind-up becomes very problematic are osteoarthritis and rheumatoid arthritis (Rowbotham, Kidd, & Porreca, 2006).

Clinical Pearl

■ Neuronal plasticity: ability of the nervous system to change or alter its function caused by continued nociceptive input

■ Wind-up: enhanced response to pain stimulus produced by prolonged pain input causing activation of the pain response in the central nervous system (D'Arcy, 2007a, 2007b)

As more has become known about the effect of pain, how pain is processed, and how pain response is formulated, there is a rich area of research that has now begun to look at what the role of genetics, gender, and race may be in how pain is perceived and processed. Although the area is still very new, the information in this chapter will provide some early insight into what is known about the differences we cannot control that affect pain modulation and medication effectiveness.

Sex, Gender, and Pain

Since the early Biblical days of Adam and Eve, who were doomed to experience physical suffering because of their errors in judgment, pain has been a topic of great discussion. How pain is produced, why it occurs, and what treatment options are effective has been discussed by both academics and average citizens. One topic that continues to be debated is the question of differences in pain sensation between men and women: Do they exist, and if so, what is causing these differences? Recent research into the difference between men's and women's pain sensations has provided some interesting information and created a need for much more research on the topic.

Do men and women experience pain differently? Yes, they do because of their hormonal variation and differences in pain pathway activation when a pain stimulus or medication is presented for interpretation. Are there differences in the way that men and women respond to pain medications? Again, the answer is yes, for a variety of reasons. Some of these differences include the following:

- Specific, different pain pathways for men and women for specific medication types
- Differences in the way pain is processed
- Effect of sex hormones
- Differences in response to opioid medications
- Differences in threshold and tolerance for pain

For many years, women were eliminated from research because it was thought that there was an estrogenic effect on pain that would skew research results. An additional consideration was the fact that estrogen levels in women fluctuated during menstrual cycles, causing data to be skewed, depending on the time of the month. Because of these suspicions, most of the early research on breast cancer was done with male subjects. Animal studies on pain were performed with desexed animals in an attempt to avoid any hormonal effect on the study results. Now, research focuses on these differences and uses them to advantage, such as in finding the causes of and treatment options for menstrual migraines.

There are some pain conditions that are more specific to women than men. Examples of these syndromes include the following:

- Fibromyalgia
- Temporomandibular pain
- Phantom breast pain
- Postmastectomy pain syndrome
- Menstrually related migraine
- Irritable bowel syndrome
- Interstitial cystitis
- Vulvodynia

In a study to compare the analgesic effect of morphine in both men and women, three important conclusions were derived:

- Morphine is more potent in women than in men.
- The onset and offset of morphine is slower in women than in men.
- Plasma concentrations of both the active drug and two metabolites were identical for both sexes (Dahan et al., 2008).

These findings are particularly important for acute pain and postoperative pain management. Because morphine is considered the gold standard for pain management medication comparison and is commonly used in postoperative pain relief, these differences in potency and onset are important considerations when pain relief is assessed. As an interesting addendum, the sex effect with morphine disappears with older patients, leading to the speculation that hormones have an effect on morphine's ability to pass through the blood-brain barrier (Dahan et al., 2008).

In addition to the differences in morphine with men and women, the side effects from opioid medications tend to have some sex-related relationships. The most common side effects with opioid medications are nausea and vomiting, sedation, cardiovascular effects, and respiratory depression. These differences include the following:

- More nausea and vomiting with women using opioids for postoperative pain control
- Increased risk of opioid-induced respiratory depression in women

- Morphine associated with lower heart rate in women but the development of hypertension in men
- With opioid use, women reported more feelings of euphoria (a high feeling) and reported more instances of dry mouth (Dahan et al., 2008)

Other differences with pain medications were related to differences seen with κ-agonist medications, such as nalbuphine, butorphanol, and pentazocine.

The melanocortin-1 receptor (MC1R) gene has a specific role in modulating a pain pathway for specific medications that exists only in women. This gene is commonly associated with people who have red hair, fair skin, freckles, and a high predisposition to melanoma (Dahan et al., 2008).

- MC1R was tested by giving pentazocine to both men and women.
- MC1R showed no pain relief in men but pain relief in women who were redheaded and fair skinned.
- The hypothesis is that men and women have separate pain pathways for processing some medications that are created by different genes and neurochemicals.

The study of differences in pain response both physiologically and to pain medications in men and women is a very new area of research. Much more research is needed to confirm these early findings. The early research is promising and points the way to finding the true differences between men and women in both pain response and medication efficacy.

Genetic Response Variability and Opioid Polymorphisms

We already know that genetics plays a big role in the production of eye color, for example. Some people can have variants of blue, green, gray, or brown eyes, based on the dominant gene expression in their individual physiology. What we are just learning is that people can also respond to opioids differently, based on their genetic makeup.

One of the most promising targets for study is the A118G single nucleotide polymorphism in the mu-opioid receptor (MOR) gene (Janicki et al., 2006; Landau, 2006). Differences in this section of genetic code are hypothesized to create differences in opioid needs and pain relief.

In a research study of patients (n = 74) who were undergoing total knee replacement, patients were genetically profiled by opioid-binding site types. Group one was AA homozygous patients who had a genetically efficient morphine metabolism pattern, group two was an AG heterozygous genetic variant, and group three was a GG homozygous nonsensitive genetic variant with reduced or impaired morphine sensitivity. The findings of morphine use via patient-controlled analgesia (PCA) and analgesia in the first 48 hours postoperatively were significantly different for both morphine consumption and pain relief:

- AA used 25 mg of morphine and had good pain relief.
- AG used 25 mg of morphine and had good pain relief.
- GG used 40 mg of morphine and had many more attempts on their PCAs trying to achieve better pain control (Chou et al., 2006).

What does this mean for the clinician? It does explain some of what we see in the clinical setting with variation in patient response to opioids. Some patients may be genetically programmed to have a good, efficient response to morphine, whereas other patients might benefit from another medication that is more suited to their genetic makeup.

In a prospective, observational study of both acute care patients (n = 101) and patients with chronic noncancer pain (n = 121), the results were somewhat different. The patients were typed either as having A118 MOR (major) or as having variant G118 MOR (minor) alleles. The results of the acute pain, postoperative group showed no statistical difference in pain scores or in morphine consumption in either group (Janicki et al., 2006). The patients with chronic pain did have some differences compared with the patients with acute pain. In the chronic pain group, the carriers of the major allele required significantly higher doses of opioids when compared with the opioid use of the patients with the minor allele (Janicki et al., 2006). This finding may reflect differences in pain processing when the NMDA receptors are activated through continued input of pain stimuli leading to neuronal plasticity.

Opioid Polymorphism: Differences in Opioid Effect Based on Genetic Differences

The variation in study results could be expected. The area of research is so new that not many replications have been performed, and study protocols are widely variant. As more research is done, there should be some consistent findings to illustrate the differences between patient groups, medications, and pain medication delivery systems (e.g., PCA versus oral).

What does this mean for clinicians? The results of the studies do seem to indicate that genetic differences can cause a patient to need more morphine to control pain. They do seem to indicate that the patients with the major gene expression (A118 MOR) had a higher need for pain medication when compared with the minor allele group (G118 MOR) if the pain was chronic. However, do genetics account for all the differences? In reality, morphine use in PCA can be a somewhat unreliable way to measure a patient's desire for using morphine for pain relief, need for medication, fear of addiction, or occurrence of side effects. If patients are nauseated, they may defer using the PCA because the pain is less burdensome than the nausea.

The biggest indication from these very basic and early studies is that there is a need for more research to better define and confirm the findings of the first studies. There is an element of excitement that the findings could really lead to a breakthrough as to why patients have such variation in response to opioids and possibly lead to the creation of a way to predetermine what type of medication or dose would be best for any patient. More research will prove or disprove these early studies and determine if we will ever be able to know what pain medication will give any patient the best pain relief.

Opioid Rotation and Equianalgesia

Many endogenous and exogenous substances, including opioids, bind to specific sites in patients' bodies. Early research identified the site for opioids binding as the mu receptor, and groups of studies to determine just how the binding was accomplished followed. As research progressed, various differences in the opioid receptors were discovered, and current research indicates that there are as many as 45 different subtypes at the mu-receptor sites (Pasternak, 2005).

Because of these variations, it is not uncommon to try one medication, have it fail, try another medication, and have it work well to relieve the patient's pain. The ability of the medication to relieve pain is truly a function of the patient's genetics and the binding ability of the medication. If the patient's best binding potential is set up for morphine, giving the patient fentanyl for pain will result in poorer outcomes and diminished pain relief.

As the binding sites become accustomed to certain pain medications, the pain relief response can be decreased. These patients report less effective pain relief with one medication after dose escalations and interval adjustment. As the doses go up, the side effect profile becomes more burdensome, so little is gained in the way of pain relief while side effects increase. In these cases, a technique called *opioid rotation* can help increase pain relief and decrease side effects, all at lower doses of a new medication.

Opioid rotation refers to the clinical practice of substituting one strong opioid for another strong opioid in an attempt to achieve a better balance between pain relief and side effects (Quigley, 2006). Another way to describe the rotation effect is switching opioids from one to another when treatment-limiting toxicity establishes poor responsiveness (Indelicato & Portnoy, 2002). Simplistically, the opioid receptor gets a little tired and overly accustomed to seeing one drug all the time and will perk up and accept (bind to) a new drug more efficiently, providing a higher level of pain relief with fewer side effects.

Which patients are candidates for opioid rotation? Chronic cancer patients who are heavily opioid dependent are excellent candidates for opioid rotation and may have a group of medications that they rotate through regularly. Chronic pain patients who have taken opioids for an extended period are also very good candidates for opioid rotation. This phenomenon was first seen in chronic pain patients when their opioid use had continued over the course of several years (Indelicato & Portnoy, 2002).

What do these patients look like clinically? These are the patients who complain of poor pain relief and continue to complain of pain with no improvement, even though the dose is escalated. In addition, as the doses continue to increase, there is a potential for side effects, such as nausea, pruritis, or other adverse reactions. The risk–benefit ratio of medication use is reached, and further dose escalation would not be useful.

In a study of patients who had cancer (n = 164), changes in opioid medication were tracked. In this patient group, 56% of the patients required opioid rotation related to side effects and ineffective pain relief. The medications being manipulated in this study were morphine, hydromorphone, methadone, fentanyl, and oxycodone (Walsh et al., 2004).

The result of opioid rotation is improved pain relief with a lower dose of medication. To perform an opioid rotation, there are several steps to follow. Using the equianalgesia conversion data (Appendix B), convert the old medication dose to a new equianalgesic dose of the new medication. Equianalgesia means equal in analgesic strength. The one warning with using this table is to remember that the doses were set in single dose studies, with opioid-naïve patients in acute care settings (Pasternak, 2005). They do not fully capture medication differences over the long term and cannot account for patient variability.

To perform the opioid rotation, calculate the correct conversion of the medication using the table, decrease the new dose by 25%–50%, and offer adequate breakthrough medication (Indelicato & Portnoy, 2002). The reduction in dose is needed because of the anticipated incomplete cross-tolerance (caused by the differences in mu receptor and binding) that leads to greater effect and increased side effects if the dose were converted at full strength (D'Arcy, 2009).

Exhibit 8.1

Opioid Rotation Conversion

Original medication: MS-Contin
MS-Contin 120 mg twice per day with MSIR 30 mg every 4 hours as needed for pain

New medication: Oxycontin
MS-Contin 120 mg twice per day (240 mg/day) is equal to Oxycontin 80 mg twice per day (160 mg/day)
MSIR 30 mg is equal to oxycodone 20 mg every 4 hours

Decrease the new dose by 25% to 50%
25% = Oxycontin 60 mg twice per day with 15 mg oxycodone
     every 4 hours for breakthrough
50% = Oxycontin 40 mg twice per day with 10 mg of oxycodone
     every 4 hours for breakthrough

Source: D'Arcy, 2009.

Additionally, the individual patient data, including comorbidities and patient age, need to be considered (Indelicato & Portnoy, 2002). Review the example in Exhibit 8.1.

There is no hard and fast rule about using morphine for breakthrough with morphine extended release or oxycodone with Oxycontin, but the Exhibit helps to show an additional conversion by also including the breakthrough option. As a prescriber, you can choose to mix and match morphine with other drugs and vice versa. The key here is to choose medications the patient has not seen in a while and to monitor the effect closely so that you can see if the change has made any difference. If you choose to go with the conservative option (50%), you can always increase the new medication up to the 25% reduction to improve pain relief if the patient starts to have increased pain. If the patient is someone who could tolerate a bigger dose, considering previous medication history, age, and comorbidities, the 25% option may work best. Always offer adequate breakthrough medication so the patient can more easily convert to the new medication regimen and retain pain control.

Other Factors

There are other factors that contribute to the use and response to opioids in the body that can also affect pain management outcomes. The liver has a group of enzymes that affect how medications are metabolized or inactivated, or provide a diminished or exaggerated response. The CYP 450 system in the liver transforms some opioids to usable metabolites. If this system is impaired or inactivated by another medication, the opioid effect will be directly affected.

Some patients have different metabolism profiles for medication utilization. If the patient has a rapid or ultrarapid medication metabolism, medication will be used quickly. These patients tell you that a standard dose of opioid medication does not last long enough. In the medication section, the warning for codeine was highlighted for rapid metabolizers because several incidents of morphine overdose were detected in infants who were nursing from mothers who had taken codeine and rapidly metabolized the codeine to morphine.

Conversely, at the other end of the spectrum, patients who metabolize medication slowly are at risk for increased effects of opioids with repeated doses. These are the patients who may say that a small dose of opioid medication lasts a long time, or they request low-dose opioids, and they may report being sensitive to opioids. These patients may also have a higher profile for oversedation, nausea and vomiting, and so forth, because the medication stays in their system for longer periods.

No matter what aspect of genetic variability you encounter in clinical practice, there are options to counteract the effect. Switching medications, trying different types of medications, or adding in coanalgesics or complementary methods may increase the potential for optimal pain relief. This is truly one area where pain management is truly an art and science, and in this case, the science is helping to facilitate the chances of finding the right medication for the individual patient.

Betsy Jones is a 45-year-old patient with chronic low back pain that she sustained in a motor vehicle accident when she was hit broadside by a drunk driver. She is fair and red headed and says that most pain medication either doesn't work or makes her feel all fuzzy headed. She rates her pain at 7/10 and says the worst part is the pain that runs down the back of her leg and feels like an electric shock. She has tried numerous opioids and nonopioid medications for pain but reports very poor pain relief.

Her primary care provider sends Betsy to you, a pain specialist, to see if there is any good answer to her pain complaint. When you examine Betsy, she has an exaggerated pain response in her lower leg to light touch. Her back pain is deep and midline in the lumbar area. You ask Betsy about other areas of her life, and she tells you, "Well, I don't sleep at all. I can't stand getting into bed and just lying there. My muscles get all crampy and achy, and my leg just burns. My husband doesn't understand. He thinks this is all in my head, and I could do better if I wanted to. The pain medications all make me feel dizzy and light-headed. When I had my back surgery, I got so sick to my stomach with the morphine that they had to stop the pain pump. I don't understand it. I only used such a little bit of medication, but I got so sick it was worse than the surgery. What can I do to make this pain better? I'm only 45 years old. I'm afraid I'll lose my husband if I can't get this pain under better control."

Questions to Consider

1. Do you suspect that Betsy's genetic profile would indicate she has some difficulty with morphine metabolism? Would you class her as a rapid, ultrarapid, moderate, slow, or ultraslow metabolizer of opioid medications?
2. What does being a fair-skinned, redheaded woman have to do with Betsy's pain management?
3. Does Betsy's gender have a role in her lack of pain relief with opioids?
4. To get a good idea of what types of medications have not worked for Betsy, she gives you a list. She has tried with only fair results, morphine (side effect: nausea and vomiting), Percocet (side effect: light-headed), Vicodin, and Tylenol #3. Would you consider trying Ultram/Ultracet, Dilaudid, or oxymorphone? Would you consider going back to one of her old medications and trying a lower dose? Would you rotate opioids?
5. What kinds of nonopioids would you suggest? Nonsteroidal anti-inflammatory drugs, acetaminophen, anticonvulsants, antidepressants, and so forth?
6. Would adding a complementary method to her pain management regimen be helpful? What would you suggest for a low back pain patient with poor pain relief and sleep dysfunction?

REFERENCES

Chou, W. Y., Yang, L. C., Lu, H. F., Ko, J. Y., Wang, C. H., Lin, S. H., . . . Hsu, C. J. (2006). Association of mu-opioid receptor gene polymorphism (A118G) with variation in morphine consumption for analgesia after total knee arthroplasty. *Acta Anaesthesiologica Scandinavica, 50*(7), 787–792.

Dahan, A., Kest, B., Waxman, A., & Sarton, E. (2008). Sex-specific response to opiates: Animal and human studies. *Anesthesia & Analgesia, 107*(1), 83–95.

D'Arcy, Y. (2007a). *Pain management: Evidence-based tools and techniques for nursing professionals.* Marblehead, MA: HCPro.

D'Arcy, Y. (2007b). One pain medication does not fit all: Using opioid rotation. *The Nurse Practitioner, 32*(11), 7–8.

D'Arcy, Y. (2009). Opioid therapy: Focus on patient safety. *American Nurse Today, 4*(5), 18–22.

Indelicato, R. A., & Portnoy, R. (2002). Opioid rotation in the management of refractory cancer pain. *Journal of Clinical Oncology, 20*(1), 348–352.

Janicki, P., Schuler, G., David, F., Bohr, A., Gordin, V., Jarzembowski, T., . . . Mets, B. (2006). A genetic association study of the functional A118G polymorphism of the human *mu*-opioid receptor gene in patients with acute and chronic pain. *Anesthesia & Analgesia, 103*(4), 1011–1017.

Landau, R. (2006). One size does note fit all: Genetic variability of muopioid receptor and postoperative morphine consumption. *Anesthesiology, 105*(2), 235–237.

Pasternak, G. W. (2005). Molecular biology of opioid analgesia. *Journal of Pain and Symptom Management, 29*(Suppl. 5), S2–S9.

Quigley, C. (2006). Opioid switching to improve pain relief and drug tolerability. *The Cochrane Database of Systemic Reviews, (3)*, CD004847.

Rowbotham, M., Kidd, B., & Porreca, F. (2006). Role of central sensitization in chronic pain: Osteoarthritis and rheumatoid arthritis compared to neuropathic pain. In H. Flor, E. Kalso, & J. Dostrovsky (Eds.), *Proceedings of the 11th World Congress on Pain*. Seattle, WA: IASP Press.

Walsh, D., Davis, M. P., Estfan, B., Legrand, S. B., Lagman, R. L., & Shaheen, P. (2004). Opioid rotation prospective longitudinal study: 8258. *Journal of Clinical Oncology, 22*(Suppl. 14), 793s.

9

Pain and Addiction

OVERVIEW

Most patients feel that when they see a health care provider for a pain complaint, a prescription for medication will be a part of the treatment. Leaving a provider's office without a prescription when pain is the reason for the visit can leave the patient feeling under-treated and misunderstood. The patient's expectations have not been met. To patients, the pain is very real, and they understand the effect it has on their daily lives. For a patient who complains of acute low back pain, being told to stay active and use Tylenol as recommended in the American Pain Society Low Back Pain Guideline may seem like the health care provider did not understand the problem as well as the patient does. Despite better outcomes, these new indications are in contrast to previous practice habits, when patients were fre-quently given medications, including opioids, for a wide variety of patient complaints.

Today, the health care provider who is providing opioid medi-cations for pain has a significant concern about providing these medications. In a survey of 400 nurse practitioners recently con-ducted in a national nurse practitioner journal, there were indica-tions of concern about the potential for addicting patients when opioids were provided, as well as fears of regulatory oversight (D'Arcy, 2009). The comfort level of the respondent practitioners

179

decreased considerably by 73% to 32% when the opioid prescribing moved from a short-term event to long-term opioid therapy for chronic pain (D'Arcy, 2009).

Today's practitioner needs to be concerned about not only providing the right medication to the right patient but also making sure that the prescribed medications are not abused, diverted, or misused. This chapter will discuss addiction, dependency, and tolerance in patients who are being seen in primary care practices. Information from several national guidelines is used to help practitioners determine when and how opioid medication can present a risk of addiction to their patients.

Prescribing Opioids

What is the current state of opioid prescribing for health care providers working in primary care practices? In a series of multisite interviews with nurse practitioners (NPs) working in primary care, pain consciousness and practice climate influenced the NPs' response to a patient's complaint of pain (Droes, 2004). The ability of the NP to understand and empathize with the patients when pain was the primary complaint affected the frequency of opioid prescriptions. NPs with high pain consciousness tended to prescribe opioids more frequently than NPs with low pain consciousness, who tended to avoid prescribing opioids (Droes, 2004).

In all 50 states, NPs have some form of prescriptive authority (American Academy of Nurse Practitioners [AANP], 2006). Most states allow NPs prescriptive authority for controlled substances at some level (AANP, 2006; D'Arcy & McCarberg, 2007). Although the opportunity for prescribing opioids to treat chronic pain is present, many NPs still have questions about what medications to use, how to prescribe opioids long term for patients with chronic pain, regulatory oversight, and legal issues. NPs struggle with these issues, and this lack of confidence affects the way opioid medications are prescribed.

Two studies (Cipher, Hooker, & Guerra, 2006; Running, Kipp, & Mercer, 2006) provided an understanding of the practice of NPs when compared with their medical colleagues. Using a retrospective 400-chart review process, Running and colleagues (2006) compared the prescribing practices of physicians and NPs in primary care practice. Prescriptions were for the treatment of an initial complaint of sinusitis, bronchitis, musculoskeletal injury, and back pain; the exposure of the NPs and physicians to patients with these conditions was similar. The findings indicate that NPs and physicians have similar prescribing patterns for patients with musculoskeletal injury and for patients with back pain. Nurse practitioner and physician prescriptions for controlled substances to treat these conditions did not differ significantly. For the non-painful conditions (sinusitis and bronchitis), NP and physician prescribing practices were also similar, with the exception of the prescription of decongestants for bronchitis, which was more frequent with NPs than with physicians (Running et al., 2006).

In another comparison study, Cipher and colleagues (2006) reviewed the National Ambulatory Medical Care Survey database, a large national database, to obtain a representative sample of 88,346 patient visits to primary care providers from 1997 to 2002. They used this information to compare prescribing patterns of physicians, physician assistants, and NPs. The average number of prescriptions (all drugs) per patient written by the three disciplines was 1.5, 1.8, and 1.7, respectively, and the percentage of prescriptions for controlled substances was 12.4%, 12.3%, and 11%, respectively; these differences were not significant (Cipher et al., 2006). Thus, the prescribing patterns for all three disciplines were remarkably similar for the number of prescriptions written overall and the number of prescriptions written for controlled substances.

Other key elements must be considered by NPs when prescribing opioids for patients. Learning to assess patients well and using tools that provide the information to enhance decision making are important additions to NP practice. It is also important to set reasonable expectations with the patient by working with the patient to determine a pain level that is acceptable to the patient, yet balances effective analgesia with possible side effects. Setting pain goals and assessing changes in functionality are fundamental to assessing progress in pain control for patients with persistent pain (American Geriatrics Society Panel on Persistent Pain in Older Persons, 2002; Marcus, 2000).

Fears of Addiction

The fear of addicting a patient when opioids are being prescribed is very real. Although studies show that NPs and other medical staff prescribe in the same patterns, NPs have real fears of addicting patients and fear regulatory oversight.

In a survey with 400 NP respondents, the NPs expressed their concerns about addicting patients and increasing the regulatory oversight of their practice. When the NP respondent group was asked about their comfort level prescribing opioids for short-term pain, 73% responded that they felt comfortable, whereas the percentage dropped to 32% when the scenario was prescribing long-term opioids for chronic low back pain (D'Arcy, 2009).

When ranking opioid-prescribing barriers, the NP respondents ranked their concerns as:

1. Cost
2. Fear of regulatory oversight
3. Addiction
4. Not knowledgeable about medications
5. Do not want to be seen as different from other prescribers (D'Arcy, 2009)

Because NPs work with many patients who are underinsured or have no insurance, the fact that cost was the first barrier identified is understandable. The second and third options, fear of regulatory oversight and addiction, indicate that a large number of the prescriber respondents do feel that addiction and investigation of prescribing practices is a real issue.

One reason the NPs cited for their concerns was a lack of preparation in their basic NP education. They indicated that the basic NP education did not prepare them to assess chronic pain (62%); treat chronic, long-term pain (44%); or choose the right medication for the pain complaint (56%) (D'Arcy, 2009). These responses indicate that approximately half of the respondents did not feel they could chose the right medication for the patient, and less than 50% indicated they were prepared to treat chronic pain.

To treat patients with chronic pain effectively, learning about chronic pain and the medications that can be used as part of the ongoing care plan is necessary. Recognizing the fears of the situation and having the knowledge base to provide care with good outcomes will boost confidence. Using national guidelines to support practice decisions is a part of providing safe care to all patient, not only to those with chronic pain. Finally, documenting all aspects of the patient's care, including the treatment agreement as discussed in Chapter 10, will provide the legal support for the prescriptive practices of the NP.

ADDICTION AND DEPENDENCE

What are the current findings about addiction and dependency? Many health care providers are still confused about the difference between dependency and addiction. They consider patients who take opioids on a daily basis to be addicted and label them as such in documentation. Many are unaware that dependency is not addiction and that the behaviors they associate with addiction may be in reality a sign of undertreated pain. Many of these patients are relief seekers, not drug seekers. Patients who take opioid medications for pain are labeled as addicted when, in truth, they are dependent on the medications. The following information should clarify the differences between the two clinical presentations.

True addiction is not as common as most health care providers think it is. The patient who knows what medication works for him or her or calls in early for a prescription may be demonstrating aberrant behaviors, but they are not addicted.

Abberant behaviors are those behaviors that are often considered to be reflective of addiction but in truth may just be an indication of undertreated pain. Some of the behaviors that are less predictive of addiction include, hoarding drugs, asking for a specific medication or dose or self escalating doses one or two times. Behaviors which seem to be more predictive of addiction are injecting oral formulations, stealing or selling drugs, and obtaining medications from non-standard sources. (Portnoy & Fine, 2004). Knowing which behaviors will be problematic can help the prescriber understand when further screening and assessment is needed. Addiction is based on the 4 C's (Table 9.1):

- Craving for the favored substance
- Compulsive use
- Lack of control over the drug
- Continued use despite harm (American Pain Society [APS], AAPM, American Society of Addiction Medicine [ASAM], 2001)

Addiction is a primary, chronic, neurobiologic disease with genetic, psychosocial, and environmental factors influencing its development and manifestations (APS, AAPM, ASAM, 2001). Addicts present to the health care provider in a very different way than other patients. Their focus is the drug of choice, and they will often have physical signs, such as track marks between toes or skin popping scars over their extremities from injecting drugs. They can also report various methods of using drugs, from injecting to skin popping, injecting oral drugs, and diversion of all types of medications. Although there have been a multitude of efforts to create a medication that cannot be misused, addicts will smoke, inject, or snort any type of opioid if it provides the physical pleasure response that they are seeking.

The one important point here is that the addict is entitled to pain relief. Many patients who are addicts are seen only through one lens, as an addict, and the pain complaints that they have are overlooked. These are very needy patients who have the right to pain

Table 9.1 ◼ *Definitions Related to Opioid Use*

Term	Definition
Addiction	A primary, chronic, neurobiologic disease, with genetic, psychosocial, and environmental factors influencing its development and manifestations. It is characterized by behaviors that include one or more of the following: ■ Impaired control over drug use ■ Compulsive use ■ Continued use despite harm ■ Craving
Physical dependence	A state of adaptation that is manifested by a drug class–specific withdrawal syndrome that can be produced by the following: ■ Abrupt cessation ■ Rapid dose reduction ■ Decreasing blood level of the drug and/or administration of an antagonist
Tolerance	A state of adaptation in which exposure to a drug induces changes that result in a diminution of one or more of the drug's effects over time
Pseudoaddiction	Patient behaviors that may occur when pain is undertreated. These may include the following: ■ Becoming focused on obtaining medications ■ "Clock watching" ■ Seemingly inappropriate "drug seeking" ■ Illicit drug use ■ Deception Unlike true addiction, pseudoaddiction resolves when the patient's pain is treated effectively

Source: American Academy of Pain Medicine, 2001. American Pain Society [APS], AAPM, American Society of Addiction Medicine [ASAM], 2001.

management but who are time consuming and very difficult to deal with in the average primary care visit. Health care prescribers cannot provide medications to a patient to continue addiction, but they can provide medications to these patients for the treatment of pain. To ensure safe prescribing practices, see the opioid agreement for documenting treatment plans and progress toward goals. The primary care practitioner should also use a variety of specialists when dealing with this type of patient to support the care they are providing. Psychologists, addicitionologists, pain specialists, social workers and counselors are just a few specialties that can assist with patients who have substance abuse issues.

Dependency, on the other hand, is a different condition when compared with addiction. All addicts are dependent on their opioids, and all patients who take opioid medications for more than 30 days are dependent. Dependency is defined as a state of adaptation that is manifested by a drug class–specific withdrawal syndrome that can be produced by the following:

- Abrupt cessation
- Rapid dose reduction
- Decreasing blood level of the drug and/or administration of an antagonist (APS, AAPM, ASAM, 2001)

The dependent patient may work and can have good family relationships. The patient who is dependent on opioid medications will use these medications to better their life, not destroy it.

It is important for the health care provider to establish a trusting relationship with the patient who has chronic pain and takes opioids regularly. Once the opioids are prescribed, there is an understanding and validation of the pain complaint and recognition on the patient's part that medication will be provided for pain relief. Respecting this understanding is important for both the patient and the prescriber. Most patients who take opioids regularly do not go on to become addicts.

Tolerance and Pseudoaddiction

Two additional conditions that are related to addiction and dependency are tolerance and pseudoaddiction. Tolerance is not a sign of addiction. A patient who takes any type of medication can become tolerant to some effect. Tolerance is simply the lessening of a medication effect over time. For example, if a patient becomes nauseated when they start a new medication, and the nausea lessens over time as the patient continues to take the medication and accommodates to it, that would be considered tolerance.

Most often, the term "tolerance" is applied to a patient when they frequently request dose increases because the medication is no longer providing the type of pain relief it once did. The lessening of the pain relief is considered to be tolerance. When patients report increased pain, it is worthwhile to ask if they are taking the medication as prescribed, if they started any new activity that might cause pain, or if they have changed the way they take the medication (e.g., before bed, in the morning, etc). The only side effect that the patient will never become tolerant to is constipation. All opioids cause constipation, and it must be treated effectively for the patient to continue to take the medication.

Once the patient reaches a stable pain state, he or she should be able to find a medication dose that controls the pain. Stable pain equates to stable medication dose. If, for some reason, this is not happening, trying to increase the dose, changing the medication interval, or using an opioid rotation strategy can help the patient retain adequate pain relief.

Pseudoaddiction is really a sign of undertreated pain. Pseudoaddiction is a condition in which the patient is perceived to be drug seeking when in reality they are relief seeking. These are the patients who are considered "drug seekers" or "clock watchers," or seem to be on the call light all the time requesting pain medication.

Behaviors that are often associated with pseudoaddiction center on the need for more pain medication. In clinical settings, when adequate pain medication is provided for these patients, the behaviors often disappear.

RECOGNIZING AND RESPONDING TO THE ADDICT WITH PAIN

No matter what substance an addict is using, they still have the right to have their pain treated. The prescriber, on the other hand, has the responsibility of safe prescribing habits and focusing on the patient's pain needs. Opioids for these patients should be given only for pain relief, and careful documentation should be done at every clinical visit and for every phone call request.

If patients are known to be abusing substances, there are some rules that can make the care of these patients a little easier to manage.

■ There should be a written treatment agreement that is discussed and signed by both the patient and provider.

■ Only one prescriber should be writing opioids for the patient.

■ The prescriber should know what other physicians that the patient sees so that all health care providers know who will be managing the patient's medications.

■ Random, observed drug screens should be done frequently, and if illicit substances or prescription medications show up, there should be clear penalties for violating the agreement.

■ If the treatment agreement is broken, the patient should be exited from any opioid prescribing but continued in the practice for treatment without opioids and treating the pain with other nonopioid medications and interventions (see Chapter 10).

Common signs of addiction include becoming more and more unkempt, injecting oral medications, stealing/forging prescriptions, performing sex for drugs, stealing drugs from others, trying to get opioids from more than one source, and buying pain medication from a street dealer (Fine & Portnoy, 2007). Behaviors that are seen as less indicative of addiction include expressing anxiety about current symptoms, hoarding medications, taking someone else's pain medication, requesting a specific drug or medication, raising dose of opioids on their own, asking for a second opinion about pain medications, drinking more alcohol when in pain, smoking cigarettes to relieve pain, and using opioids to treat other symptoms (Fine & Portnoy, 2007). Of the total pain clinic population using opioids for pain relief, 40% will exhibit aberrant behaviors, 20% will abuse/misuse their medications, and 2%–5% will become addicted. Although this population is not typical, it does give us a picture of a group of patients who are exposed to high usages of opioid medications.

Many health care providers are reluctant to ask these personal types of questions. It is important to know if the patient is drinking as an adjunct method for pain relief. Because alcohol is cheap and easy to get, alcohol can be combined with pain medications to help augment the effect of the prescribed medications, but it significantly increases the risk of sedation and respiratory depression.

For all health care providers working with patients with chronic pain, it is essential to become comfortable with asking the hard questions. It is also critical that, when the patient responds honestly, they are treated with a nonjudgmental approach. One way to address this is to tell the patient you are not truly interested in all of the drug-taking behaviors, but that you need to know what he or she is taking or using so that you can treat the pain more effectively. Patients with a history of substance abuse or who are actively using illicit substances will require higher doses of medication than patients with similar injuries who are not using other drugs, and the patients without a history of substance abuse will not have the same dose requirements as the patient who is addicted to an opioid substance. Over time the patient has become more sensitive to pain but less responsive to medications used to treat pain.

The primary care practitioner may not be aware that the patient they have started to treat is an addict. In this case, once the addiction is detected, using a team of specialists can help the provider give the patient adequate care while being supported by a team of experts in the area.

You are assigned to Sara Peters, 35, who is coming in to see you with complaints of neck pain for a motor vehicle accident two years ago. Sara was intoxicated and hit a telephone pole, and she sustained a whiplash injury to her neck and ruptured several cervical discs. She is not a surgical candidate and needs to have pain relief. You ask her who she has been seeing for her pain management needs and she tells you, "Really, I just need some Percocet is all. My last doctor said I couldn't have any more, and so I really need to find someone who can help me with this pain and Percocet seems to do the best job. The last doctor said I was addicted to the pills and wanted me to try other types of pain medication. I can't sleep unless I have my Percocet, and I need to sleep to be able to go to work."

When you ask her about other drugs she says, "Well yeah, I used to smoke marijuana and did some cocaine when I was younger, but now I don't have the money to buy drugs and I don't have the urge." She has copies of her most recent radiographic studies that show ruptured cervical vertebrae at several levels.

How are you going to treat Sara's pain?

> ### Questions to Consider
>
> 1. Is Sara addicted or dependent on her Percocet? Does she exhibit behaviors that are more or less predictive of addiction?
> 2. Does she have a source of pain? If so what is the best approach to treat it? Short-acting pain medications, such as Percocet, or an extended-release medication?
> 3. Is she drug seeking?
> 4. Do you feel comfortable giving Sara opioids for pain? Are there other options you could try for pain relief?
> 5. What types of protective measure can you take to ensure that the medications you give Sara are not diverted?

REFERENCES

American Academy of Nurse Practitioners. (2006). *AANP 2006 Membership Survey.* Retrieved from http://www.aanp.org/NR/rdonlyres/809B1FD3-209D-43C7-8375-C24E0744318A/0/2006MembershipSurvey.pdf

American Academy of Pain Medicine, American Pain Society, & American Society of Addiction Medicine. (2001). Definitions related to the use of opioids for the treatment of pain. Retrieved from http://www.painmed.org/productpub/statements/pdfs/definition.pdf

American Geriatrics Society Panel on Persistent Pain in Older Persons. (2002). The management of persistent pain in older persons. *Journal of the American Geriatrics Society, 50*(Suppl. 6), S205–S224.

Cipher, D. J., Hooker, R. S., & Guerra, P. (2006). Prescribing trends by nurse practitioners and physician assistants in the United States. *Journal of the American Academy of Nurse Practitioners, 18,* 291–296.

D'Arcy, Y. (2009). Be in the know about pain management. *The Nurse Practitioner, 34*(4), 43–47.

D'Arcy, Y., & McCarberg, B. (2007). NP prescribing authority for opioids. *Pain Medicine News, 5*(1), 25–26.

Droes, N. S. (2004). Role of the nurse practitioner in managing patients with pain. *Internet Journal of Advanced Nursing Practice, 6.* Retrieved from http://www.ispub.com/ostia/index.php?xmlPrinter=true&xmlFilePath=journals/ijanp/vol6n2/pain.xml

Marcus, D. A. (2000). Treatment of nonmalignant chronic pain. *American Family Physician, 61*, 1331–1336.

Running, A., Kipp, C., & Mercer, V. (2006). Prescriptive patterns of nurse practitioners and physicians. *Journal of the American Academy of Nurse Practitioners, 18*, 228–233.

ADDITIONAL RESOURCES

Adriaensen, H., Vissers, K., Noorduin, H., & Meert, T. (2003). Opioid tolerance and dependence: an inevitable consequence of chronic treatment? *Acta Anaesthesiologica Belgica, 54*, 37–47.

American Pain Foundation. (2005). *Pain facts. An overview of American pain surveys.* Retrieved from http://www.painfoundation.org/page .asp?file=Library/PainSurveys.htm

American Pain Society. (2000). *Pain assessment and treatment in the managed care environment. A position statement from the American Pain Society.* Glenview, IL: Author.

American Pain Society. (2003). *Principles of analgesic use in the treatment of acute pain and cancer pain* (5th ed.). Glenview, IL: Author.

American Pain Society. (2005). *APS glossary of pain terminology.* Retrieved from http://www.ampainsoc.org/links/pain_glossary.htm

American Pain Society. (2007). *A joint statement from the 21 Health Organizations and the Drug Enforcement Administration. Promoting pain relief and preventing abuse of pain medications: A critical balancing act.* Retrieved from http://www.ampainsoc.org/advocacy/pdf/ consensus_1.pdf

Berry, P. H., Katz, J. A., Covington, E. C., Miaskowski, C., Dahl, J. L., & American Pain Society. (2006). *Pain: Current understanding of assessment, management, and treatments.* Reston, VA: National Pharmaceutical Council.

D'Arcy, Y. M. (2007). *Pain management: Evidence-based tools and techniques for nursing professionals.* Marblehead, MA: HCPro.

D'Arcy, Y., & McCarberg, B. (2005). Field guide to pain: Developing a plan of care. *Nurse Practitioner, 30*, 60–62.

D'Arcy, Y., & McCarberg, B. (2006). Physician–nurse practitioner collaboration. *Pain Medicine News, 4*, 1, 10.

Joranson, D. E. (1995). Intractable pain treatment laws and regulations. *American Pain Society Bulletin, 5*, 1–3, 15–17.

Joranson, D. E., Ryan, K. M., Gilson, A. M., & Dahl, J. L. (2000). Trends in medical use and abuse of opioid analgesics. *JAMA: The Journal of the American Medical Association, 283*, 1710–1714.

Lazarus, J. B., & Downing, B. (2003). Monitoring and investigating certified registered nurse practitioners in pain management. *The Journal of Law, Medicine & Ethics: A Journal of the American Society of Law, Medicine & Ethics, 31*, 101–118.

United States Drug Enforcement Administration. (2001). *Prescription pain medications: Frequently asked questions and answers for health care professionals, and law enforcement personnel.* Retrieved from http://www.aapsonline.org/painman/deafaq.pdf

USA Today, & Sternberg, S. (2005). *Chronic pain: The enemy within.* Retrieved from http://www.usatoday.com/news/health/2005–05-08-chronic-pain-cover_x.htm

10

Developing a Comprehensive Treatment Plan for Patients With Chronic Pain

OVERVIEW

As with all treatment options, there is a risk–benefit analysis that should take place before the option to treat the patient's complaint is chosen. When the main treatment focus is chronic pain and opioids are being considered, the analysis must take a wider view that incorporates all aspects of the patient's lifestyle. In today's press, the issue of undertreated chronic pain is becoming a frequent topic of conversation and debate. On the other hand, the information on increasing opioid abuse, misuse, and prescription fraud provides a counterbalance to the discussion. Where does this leave the primary care prescriber who cares for the majority of these patients?

As discussed previously in this book, there are barriers that prevent health care practitioners from prescribing opioids. For nurse practitioners (NPs), some major concerns with traditional (scheduled) opioid use in the treatment of chronic pain include the fear of physical dependence and addiction, which may result in the underusage of opioid analgesics, use of non-opioid analgesics when opioids are indicated as with severe level pain, and in prescriptions written at suboptimal doses. In addition, fears regarding legal ramifications of prescribing long-term opioid therapy may be allayed by recent reports showing the low risk of Drug Enforcement Administration (DEA) sanctions. In fiscal year 2003, 50 physicians (0.005% of all physicians registered) were arrested for activities that were knowingly and intentionally beyond the scope of medical practice. Administrative sanctions, as opposed to criminal investigations, are used for allegations of faulty record keeping, and in fiscal year 2003, 67 such actions occurred. There is no record of any litigation against an NP involving controlled substances or prescribing practices although there has been a case of voluntary surrender of a license by an NP involving prescribing of controlled substances. In addition, state laws and policies regarding opioid use are showing a trend toward adopting laws or guidelines that specifically recognize the use of opioids to treat intractable pain. Intractable pain treatment acts have been established in some states and are being established in others.

The newest recommendation by the U.S. Food and Drug Administration (FDA) is the requirement that drug companies provide risk management sheets, also known as a Risk Evaluation and Mitigation Strategy, for all opioids. These documents will provide a good risk–benefit assessment for many of the most common opioids and will help prescribers determine which medication will provide the best pain relief with the lowest risk profile. These documents should be available when they are developed on the FDA website. Currently the FDA has rejected some early attempts at REM development for opioids and revision to the documents is in process.

There are techniques and practices that can provide an element of comfort for health care providers prescribing long-term opioids for treating painful chronic conditions. For these patients and providers, setting up safe prescribing practices and using opioid agreements to clarify the goals and expectations of opioid use is good practice. The following section will describe safe prescribing practices and provide examples of screening tools and documentation forms that can assist with providing a safe environment for opioids prescribing.

SAFE PRESCRIBING

- Would you sign a blank prescription and have another provider fill it in?
- Would you give a patient a post dated prescription?
- Would you give a patient a sequential set of prescriptions to be used at a future date?

If you answered yes to any of these questions, you should reconsider your prescribing practices. All of these practices could result in prosecution and loss of licensure. All of these options leave the door open to prescription misuse and abuse.

Clinical Pearl	Elements of a safe prescription for opioids:

- Date of issue
- Patient's name and address
- Practitioner's name, address, and DEA registration number
- Drug name, strength, dosage form
- Quantity prescribed
- Direction for use
- Number of refills
- Manual signature of prescriber

There is one factor that will remain constant for health care providers who treat chronic pain. Opioids will need to be used at some point for some patients. Learning the correct methods for safe opioid prescribing, such as safe prescription writing, will help the prescribing practitioner feel more comfortable with the process.

Opioids have been considered as a viable option for effective treatment of chronic pain for many years (American Academy of Pain Medicine & American Pain Society, 1997). When opioids are used to treat pain, the majority of patients taking the opioids do not become addicted. However, it has become increasing apparent that there is some risk of addiction in the general primary care patient population. How big the risk is cannot be fully determined with the current literature database. Some of the best data indicate that the risk of real addiction is low, <5% or 2%–5% of pain clinic patients. Even the best research in this area does not provide a definitive answer to the question of addiction in a general patient population.

There are some indications that the problem is real and increasing in significance. As the use of opioids increased (as of 2002 it is estimated that 4 to 6 million American patients were receiving opioids), 12% of all medications prescribed in ambulatory care office visits were noted to be opioids. During the same period, admission to substance abuse centers for narcotic (opioid) painkillers increased by 155% between 1992 and 2002, and the number of emergency room visits for narcotic (opioid) analgesic abuse increased 117% from 1994 to 2002.

The Substance Abuse and Mental Health Services Administration reported in a 2007 survey that 6.9 million persons used prescription drugs that were classified as psychotherapeutic in the past month, with opioids making up 5.2 million usages. Prescription drug abuse among teens has been steadily increasing over the past decade, despite advertisement campaigns to make parents and pharmacies aware of the dangers. Between the years 1992 and 2002, new opioid users increased by 542%; for college students, from 1993 to 2005, the number who reported opioid use in the past month increased by 343%. Despite these sobering statistics that indicate prescriptions are being misused, rates of addiction are not increasing by anywhere near the number indicated by the abuse statistics.

In one of the most recent findings, the incidence of addiction in a meta-analysis was 0.19% for a preselected group of patients who had never been exposed to opioids and 3.27% for a preselected group of patients who had a history of opioid abuse or addiction (Fishbain et al., 2008). In another study of 800 primary care patients being treated for a variety of pain complaints, the incidence of addiction for the overall group was found to be similar to other studies, where the addiction rate was between 4% and 6% (Flemming et al., 2007). In an analysis of addiction studies assessing the prevalence of addiction in chronic pain patients, the rates of addiction were found to be similar to the general population. This means that the vast majority of primary care patients in the studies were using their opioid medications correctly, with a select few developing true addiction.

In light of these findings, prescribers who are providing opioids for patients need to adopt practices that can protect prescribers from any inquiries into prescribing practices or regulatory review. Safe prescribing simply means that prescribing practices follow current national guideline recommendations, legal requirements, and use standard techniques for screening and continuing opioid therapy for patients who require long-term medication therapy. Using safe prescribing practice protects both the prescriber and the patient.

Screening tools are used when starting the patients on opioid therapy to determine the level of risk, if a patient on opioids is having difficulty managing the opioid therapy, and continued screening of the patient on opioid therapy is used to determine if aberrant behaviors are developing. Random urine screens are incorporated into the opioid treatment agreement that patients on opioid therapy should sign prior to initiation of long-term opioid therapy. The combination of urine screening, opioid treatment agreements, and screening tools should always be used together and not as a solo measure of risk assessment.

Clinical Pearl

What is a safe prescription?

- A risk–benefit ratio analysis is included before a medication is prescribed for a patient.
- Screening tools and diagnostics are used to help determine if the medication is a safe choice for the patient.
- A clear readable prescription with clear directions for use is provided.
- The right drug in the right dose for the right patient.

LEGALITIES OF OPIOID PRESCRIBING

The fear of increased regulatory oversight also colors the way a prescriber provides opioid medications for pain. If prescribers has a high fear level, they can be tempted to use less effective medications to treat pain in their patients. Findings from a survey with 963,385 registered physicians found that when adequate documentation exists in the medical records, the risk of action against any physician who prescribes opioids for chronic pain is very small.

What the survey did reveal, however, is that of the large group of physicians cited previously, there were 47 arrests in 2003. In addition, there were 56 DEA revocations from 2003 and 2004. Most of the physicians in the legal actions did not have a primary patient–physician relationship that would merit continued opioid prescribing. Some of the reasons for legal action included:

- Prescriber substance abuse
- Fraud
- Loss of medical license
- Sex in exchange for prescriptions
- Prescribing without seeing the patient

In another review of press reports of trials or indictments, opioid prescribing offences were tracked from 2004 to 2005. In this group of 47 cases with 53 physicians, 32 of the cases involved the prescribing of opioids to persons outside of legitimate medical practice. Only two of the cases were reviewed by state medical boards before the cases were initiated. These public reports of physician wrongdoing without adequate review can contribute strongly to provider fears of oversight and legal review.

Most states have laws that govern opioid prescribing, and the federal government requires a license to prescribe opioids. These requirements lend themselves to tracking the prescriptive practices of physicians, nurse practitioners, and physician's assistants. When considering the overall picture, it is wise to consider that of all the thousands of physicians practicing and prescribing opioids in the United States in 2002, only 120 were sanctioned by state medical boards and many had multiple violations. The findings of a review of state medical board sanctioning practice found that if the physician had an intact patient–physician relationship and the opioids were documented for treating a painful condition, the risk of formal sanction was very low.

Although pictures of health care providers being taken off to jail or news releases about prescribers being sanctioned for prescription abuse with opioids make headlines and leave a lasting impression, they should always be considered in light of the true findings. Most health care providers follow prescribed rules and regulations for prescribing opioids. If proper documentation accompanies these practices, the risk of legal intervention is seen to be very low.

UNIVERSAL PRECAUTIONS

Standardized guidelines have been suggested to manage all patients with chronic pain. By utilizing this approach, clinicians can lower the risks associated with opioid administration. These guidelines have been termed *universal precautions in pain management*, borrowing the concept of "universal precautions" from the infectious disease model, suggesting that it not possible for clinicians to assess all risks associated with opioid therapy (Gourlay, Heit, & Almahrezi, 2005). Therefore, it is appropriate to apply the minimum level of precaution to all patients utilizing this treatment. A more complete description of these precautionary steps is provided in this and other chapters of this book. The following steps from these guidelines are as follows:

- Make a diagnosis with an appropriate differential
- Psychological assessment, including risk of addictive disorders
- Informed consent
- Treatment agreement
- Pre- and postintervention assessment of pain level and function
- Appropriate trial of opioid therapy with or without adjunctive medication
- Reassessment of pain score and level of function
- Regularly assess the four As of pain medicine (analgesic, activities of daily living, adverse effects, and aberrant behaviors)
- Periodically review pain diagnosis and comorbid conditions, including addictive disorders
- Documentation that is complete and addresses all elements of assessment, medications, and treatment indications such as pain.

USING SCREENING TOOLS

Screening tools can provide a good baseline for monitoring patient behaviors, detecting aberrant behaviors, and determining the risk of long-term opioid therapy. Most patients in pain clinics will undergo a screening process that includes an opioid screening tool when long-term opioid therapy is being considered as an option. Some patients exhibit aberrant behaviors that can skew the health care provider's willingness to continue with opioid medications. Using tools to monitor the appearance and meaning related to the risk potential for using opioids will help the practitioner decide if opioid therapy for an individual patient has a favorable risk–benefit ratio.

Some of the simplest screens are the CAGE and the TRAUMA screen. The CAGE questions include:

- Have you ever tried to *c*ut down on your alcohol or drug use?
- Have people *a*nnoyed you by commenting on or critiquing your drinking or drug use?
- Have you ever felt bad or *g*uilty about your drinking or drug use?
- Have you ever needed and *e*ye opener first thing in the morning to steady your nerves or get rid of a hangover?

The higher the number of positive responses, the greater the likelihood that the patient has a drug or alcohol abuse problem.

In the TRAUMA screen, the person's injury profile is assessed. To perform this screen the patient is asked the following questions.

Since your 18th birthday, have you:

- Had any fractures or dislocations to your bones or joints (excluding sports injuries)?
- Been injured in a traffic accident?
- Injured your head (excluding sports injuries)?
- Been in a fight or assaulted while intoxicated?
- Been injured while intoxicated?

If the patient has a positive response to two or more of the questions in the TRAUMA screen, there is a high potential for abuse.

For any of these simple screens, if there is concern about the potential for addiction, medication misuse, or the development of addictive behaviors, using the more complex screens listed subsequently can help identify the magnitude of risk if opioid therapy is being considered. The more complex screens are as follows:

1. *Screener and Opioid Assessment for Patients with Pain* assesses for abuse potential using a 14-item self-report measure. This is a reliable and valid measure where a score of equal to or greater than 8 indicates a high risk of misuse or abuse.

Exhibit 10.1

Date _____

Patient Name _____

OPIOID RISK TOOL

		Mark each box that applies	Item Score If Female	Item Score If Male
1. Family History of Substance Abuse	Alcohol	[ ]	1	3
	Illegal Drugs	[ ]	2	3
	Prescription Drugs	[ ]	4	4
2. Personal History of Substance Abuse	Alcohol	[ ]	3	3
	Illegal Drugs	[ ]	4	4
	Prescription Drugs	[ ]	5	5
3. Age (Mark box if 16 – 45)		[ ]	1	1
4. History of Preadolescent Sexual Abuse		[ ]	3	0
5. Psychological Disease	Attention Deficit Disorder	[ ]	2	2
	Obsessive Compulsive Disorder			
	Bipolar			
	Schizophrenia			
	Depression	[ ]	1	1
TOTAL		[ ]		

Total Score Risk Category	Low Risk 0 – 3	Moderate Risk 4 – 7	High Risk ≥ 8

Source: Used with permission of the author.

2. *Opioid Risk Tool* screens for aberrant behaviors in patients on long-term opioids using a five-item yes/no format self-report measure. Scores of 0–3 are considered low risk, 4–7 are considered moderate risk, and 8 and over are considered high risk. It has an excellent ability to differentiate low-risk from high-risk patients in both men and women (Exhibit 10.1).

3. *Diagnosis, Intractability, Risk, and Efficacy Score* is a clinician-rated scale with questions in four categories: diagnosis, intractability, risk, and efficacy. The categories are further divided into psychological, chemical health, reliability, and social support. A score of 14 and above indicates a patient is a good risk for opioid therapy and those with lower scores are not considered good risks for opioid therapy.

4. *Current Opioid Misuse Measure (COMM)* is a 17-item self-report measure to identify aberrant drug-related behaviors for patients on long-term opioid therapy. The COMM is a newer tool that can identify emotional/psychiatric issues, evidence of lying, appointment patterns, and medication misuse/noncompliance (Passik, Kirsh, & Casper, 2008). Copies of these tools are available at www.painedu.com

There are many other tools that can be used to screen patients for opioid misuse and aberrant behaviors, and evaluate risk with opioid use. The above tools are those that are being used most consistently in the current clinical settings.

OPIOID AGREEMENT

Opioid treatment agreements delineate the basis for a therapeutic trial of opioid analgesics. Expectations and obligations of both the patient and the clinician are explained and put into writing. Boundaries are set for continued use of these medications while providing an opportunity for early identification and intervention of aberrant behaviors.

An agreement can be used as an educational document explaining the expectations of treatment, establishing the patient–practitioner relationship, and enhancing compliance. Elements of the agreement vary in content, but generally include:

■ Risks and benefits of treatment
■ Goals of treatment
■ Side effects of medications
■ Definitions of addiction, dependence, and tolerance
■ Rationale for changing or discontinuing medication
■ Expected patient behaviors

Examples of expected patient behaviors include the following: only take the prescriptions as directed, do not use alcohol or other sedating medications while taking opioids unless directed by your practitioner, receive opioid prescriptions only from the prescriber(s) listed, have the prescription filled only at one pharmacy, and do not request prescription refills early. Examples of opioid treatment agreements can be found at www.npweb.org or at the website for the American Academy of Pain Medicine (Exhibit 10.2).

It should be noted that the use of an opioid treatment agreement is one of several tools to monitor adherence. The act of signing the agreement is not a fail-safe preventative measure for subsequent prescription opioid abuse, and repeated review of the terms of the agreement is advisable.

When a patient deviates from the treatment agreement, the clinician must decide on an appropriate course of action. Although there is no clear-cut standard practice, several options may be considered based on the degree of departure and circumstances surrounding the incident. Options may include discharging the patient from the practice but continuing to treat the patient without opioid analgesics, continuing to treat the patient with greater vigilance, or referring the patient to a pain specialist or addictionologist. The decision must be based on a thorough assessment, with documentation of treatment rationale. The practitioner should not continue the same treatment without a thorough assessment, and documentation. If the decision is made to discharge the patient from the practice, a discussion with the patient as to the circumstances that led to this decision must take place. An addictions specialist or pain specialist should be included in the discussion of directions for opioid weaning, management of withdrawal side effects, and referral to an alternate provider, with accompanying documentation (D'Arcy & Bruckenthal, 2011).

HOW TO USE URINE SCREENING RESULTS

The frequency of urine screening should be determined by office policy and patient risk. Most clinics initially test all patients who are starting on opioid therapy and then test intermittently throughout the course of their treatment. Clinicians may identify a patient at greater risk for misuse as determined by the Pain Assessment and Documentation Tool (PADT), COMM, or aberrant behaviors.

Exhibit 10.2

SAMPLE OPIOID TREATMENT AGREEMENT

Patient Name:_____   Date:_____

Opioid (narcotic) treatment for chronic pain is used to reduce pain and improve what you are able to do each day. Along with opioid treatment, other medical care may be prescribed to help improve your ability to do daily activities. This may include exercise, use of non-narcotic analgesics, physical therapy, psychological counseling or other therapies or treatment. Vocational counseling may be provided to assist in your return to work effort.

To the doctor: Keep signed originals in your file; give a photocopy to the patient. Renew at least every 6 months.

I, _____, understand that compliance with the following guidelines is important in continuing pain treatment with Dr. _____.

1. I understand that I have the following responsibilities:
   a. I will take medications only at the dose and frequency prescribed.
   b. I will not increase or change medications without the approval of this doctor.
   c. I will actively participate in RTW efforts and in any program designed to improve function (including social, physical, psychological and daily or work activities).
   d. I will not request opioids or any other pain medicine from physicians other than from this doctor. This doctor will approve or prescribe all other mind and mood altering drugs.
   e. I will inform this doctor of all other medications that I am taking.
   f. I will obtain all medications from one pharmacy, when possible known to this doctor with full consent to talk with the pharmacist given by signing this agreement.
   g. I will protect my prescriptions and medications. Only one lost prescription or medication will be replaced in a single calendar year. I will keep all medications from children.
   h. I agree to participate in psychiatric or psychological assessments, if necessary.

   i. If I have an addiction problem, I will not use illegal or street drugs or alcohol. This doctor may ask me to follow through with a program to address this issue. Such programs may include the following:
      ■ 12-step program and securing a sponsor
      ■ Individual counseling
      ■ Inpatient or outpatient treatment
      ■ Other: _____

2. I understand that in the event of an emergency, this doctor should be contacted and the problem will be discussed with the emergency room or other treating physician. I am responsible for signing a consent to request record transfer to this doctor. No more than 3 days of medications may be prescribed by the emergency room or other physician without this doctor's approval.

3. I understand that I will consent to random drug screening. A drug screen is a laboratory test in which a sample of my urine or blood is checked to see what drugs I have been taking.

4. I will keep my scheduled appointments and/or cancel my appointment a minimum of 24 hours prior to the appointment.

5. I understand that this doctor may stop prescribing opioids or change the treatment plan if:
   a. I do not show any improvement in pain from opioids or my physical activity has not improved.
   b. My behavior is inconsistent with the responsibilities noted in #1 above.
   c. I give, sell or misuse the opioid medications.
   d. I develop rapid tolerance or loss of improvement from the treatment.
   e. I obtain opioids from other than this doctor.
   f. I refuse to cooperate when asked to get a drug screen.
   g. If an addiction problem is identified as a result of prescribed treatment or any other addictive substance.
   h. If I am unable to keep follow-up appointments.

_____   _____   _____   _____
Patient Signature   Date   Physician Signature   Date

SAMPLE OPIOID TREATMENT AGREEMENT *(continued)*

YOUR SAFETY RISKS WHILE WORKING UNDER THE INFLUENCE OF OPIOIDS:

You should be aware of potential side effects of opioids such as decreased reaction time, clouded judgment, drowsiness and tolerance. Also, you should know about the possible danger associated with the use of opioids while operating heavy equipment or driving.

SIDE EFFECTS OF OPIOIDS:
- Confusion or other change in thinking abilities
- Problems with coordination or balance that may make it unsafe to operate dangerous equipment or motor vehicles
- Breathing too slowly – overdose can stop your breathing and lead to death
- Nausea
- Constipation
- Sleepiness or drowsiness
- Aggravation of depression
- Vomiting
- Dry mouth

THESE SIDE EFFECTS MAY BE MADE WORSE IF YOU MIX OPIOIDS WITH OTHER DRUGS, INCLUDING ALCOHOL.

RISKS:
- Physical dependence. This means that abrupt stopping of the drug may lead to withdrawal symptoms characterized by one or more of the following:

Runny nose	Difficulty sleeping for several days
Diarrhea	Abdominal cramping
Sweating	'Goose bumps'
Rapid heart rate	Nervousness

- Psychological dependence. This means it is possible that stopping the drug will cause you to miss or crave it.
- Tolerance. This means you may need more and more drug to get the same effect.
- Addiction. A small percentage of patients may develop addiction problems based on genetic or other factors.
- Problems with pregnancy. If you are pregnant or contemplating pregnancy, discuss with your physician.

PAYMENT OF MEDICATIONS:

State law forbids L&I from paying for opioids once the patient reaches maximum medical improvement. You and your doctor should discuss other sources of payment for opioids when L&I can no longer pay.

RECOMMENDATIONS TO MANAGE YOUR MEDICATIONS:

- Keep a diary of the pain medications you are taking, the medication dose, time of day you are taking them, their effectiveness and any side effects you may be having.
- Use of a medication box that you can purchase at your pharmacy that is already divided into the days of the week and times of the day so it is easier to remember when to take your medications.
- Take along only the amount of medicine you need when leaving home so there is less risk of loosing all your medications at the same time.

I have read this document, understand and have had all my questions answered satisfactorily. I consent to the use of opioids to help control my pain and I understand that my treatment with opioids will be carried out as described above.

Patient Signature	Date	Physician Signature	Date

Under these circumstances, more frequent urine testing is indicated. It may be more convenient in certain office settings to set a standard of screening everyone on opioid therapy every 3 months but other settings may be better suited to a longer period of time. However, if a patient has deviated from the opioid agreement, and a decision based on the magnitude of the deviation is made to continue opioid therapy, more frequent urine testing is advised.

Testing procedures vary from laboratory to laboratory. A laboratory that performs a two-step urine screen is recommended. The first step is a screen for the general classification of compounds using enzyme immunoassay. The second step is a confirmatory process using a method of gas chromatography/mass spectrometry (GC/MS). This step detects the presence of specific compounds within the class.

Results of the urine drug screen should be used to improve patient care; therefore, careful interpretation of results in concert with other methods of assessment should be used in decision making. A positive urine drug test result is defined as:

- The prescribed drug not present
- Presence of an unprescribed opioid
- The presence of an illicit substance

The issues of cross-reactivity and false-positives and -negatives need to be considered. For example:

- Several quinolone antibiotics can potentially produce false-positive results for opioids by immunoassay, but are not misidentified by GC/MS.
- codeine and heroin metabolizes to morphine, so both substances may be identified in urine following codeine or heroin use, resulting in a false-positive for morphine.
- hydrocodone can be metabolized to hydromorphone.
- Marijuana is not usually detected in the urine from passive smoke inhalation.
- Marijuana can be detected in urine after cessation of use for up to 80 days in heavy users.
- Cocaine may be present in urine for 2 to 3 days if used as a topical anesthetic in dental or other procedures, and medical records should confirm this.

- Coca leaf teas can produce false-positive results for Cocaine.
- Poppy seed is the only substance that can cause a false-positive opioid result in GC/MS (cakes, bagels, muffins, rolls, and Danish pastry may contain poppy seeds).
- Vicks nasal inhaler, selegiline, and some diet pills can cause a false-positive for amphetamines.
- Heroin is difficult to detect because of a half-life of 5–30 minutes, resulting in false-negatives.
- A small percentage of patients metabolize opioids, especially oxycodone, rapidly resulting in a false-negative for this drug (Bruckenthal, 2007).

Urine drug screens are useful tools in a comprehensive opioid monitoring program, but clinicians are urged to consider possible discrepancies in interpretation of results prior to treatment decision making. Consider the possibilities that the patient may not have recently used the medication, the patient is a rapid metabolizer, or the test was not sensitive enough to detect concentrations or lab/clerical errors. In these instances, a second urine drug screen may be needed for clarification. Most concerning is the absence of the prescribed opioid, which may represent diversion of the drug. If the explanation for the positive urine screen does not seem reasonable, discharge from the clinic may be warranted to reduce the risk of drug diversion.

DOCUMENTING WITH THE PADT

The PADT is a specialized chart note designed to aid clinicians in monitoring outcomes during long-term therapy for noncancer patients on opioid therapy. It takes only minutes to complete and should supplement existing documentation. The elements of the four A's are the foundation of the tool, and a final section requires the interpretation of the data to formulate an assessment of the risks (e.g., side effects) and benefits (e.g., pain relief, improved functioning) of continued therapy and designation of the analgesic plan (e.g., continued therapy, dose adjustment, discontinuation). Pilot testing of the PADT demonstrated that patients on long-term opioid therapy achieved relatively positive outcomes in terms of analgesia, functionality, and tolerable side effects. Potential aberrant behaviors were common but viewed as indicator of a problem in only 10% of the cases.

The elements of this 2-page follow-up assessment tool include the following:

■ Current analgesic regime
■ Level of analgesia: average, worst, amount of pain relief from medications
■ Activities of daily living: physical, family, and social relationships, mood, and sleep
■ Adverse events
■ Potential drug-related behaviors
■ Clinician assessment/impression of the opioid therapy
■ Specific plan (Copies of the PADT can be obtained from the Jannssen Pharma website.)

CHRONIC OPIOID THERAPY GUIDELINES

When the prescriber initiates opioid therapy, there are guidelines and standards that can help provide support for the practice and provide direction for appropriate prescribing. Some of the most commonly used guidelines include the following:

■ **Department of Defense clinical practice guidelines for the management of opioid therapy for chronic pain. Retrieved from www.guideline.gov (2003).**
This guideline makes recommendations for opioid therapy for chronic pain, comprehensive assessment, pain assessment, contraindications to opioid therapy, indications for referral, and patient education. Additionally, it recommends the development and documentation of a treatment plan, consent for opioid therapy, and the use of the four A's of reassessment. It also discusses what to do with patients who do not adhere to their opioid agreement.
■ **Opioids in the management of chronic noncancer pain: An update of American Society of the Interventional Pain Physicians (ASIPP) guidelines. Retrieved from www.painphysicianjournal.com (2008).**
A detailed list of practice recommendations is made with levels of research being rated. Practice recommendations include deferment of opioids if at all possible in pregnant patients, the prescribing of

methadone by clinically expert practitioners, using a complete history and physical at the onset of therapy, the use of opioids rotations, and monitoring parameters.

■ **Clinical guidelines for the use of long-term opioid therapy in chronic noncancer pain (sponsored by the American Pain Society and the American Academy of Medicine). Retrieved from www.sciencedirect.com (2009).**
A guideline developed by a panel of members of the ASIPP. Recommendations include that opioids are effective for reducing pain and improving functional status in the short-term, that they are questionable in the long-term, and discusses issues of misuse and opioid abuse.

■ **Assessment and management of chronic pain. Retrieved from www.guideline.gov (2008).**
Encourages patient-centered care, endorses a comprehensive assessment process, argues that medications should not be the sole focus of treatment, and monitoring for opioids misuse and abuse is encouraged. A healthy lifestyle is encouraged.

■ **Pharmacological management of persistent pain in older persons. Retrieved from the American Geriatrics Society website (2009).**
A new update of an older version of the position statement by the American Geriatrics Society. Practice recommendations include discouraging the use of nonsteroidal anti-inflammatory drugs in older patients, weak evidence but a strong recommendation to use opioids is provided, and combinations of nonopioids or addition of nonopioids, such as muscle relaxants, is defined.

To protect clinical practice when prescribing opioids, it is important to take the time to set up an opioid agreement, do a complete and comprehensive history and physical examination, and establish a baseline pain screen for all patients. Using a team approach with a variety of specialists such as pain specialists, addicitionologists, psychologists and other disciplines who have an expertise in treating addiction and patients with substance abuse issues can support the primary care practitioner treating a patient with long term opioids. Having the correct documentation to indicate the use of the medications is the best defense, in case of any questions about prescribing practice.

Case Study

When you see James Jones for the first time, he tells you he needs Oxycontin to control his pain because all the other medications don't work for him. James is a 36-year-old construction worker who was injured in a work-related fall that left him with neck and back pain. He has been seen by the physical medicine and rehabilitation clinic, and they cannot work with him because he complains that his pain is too severe and radiates down both his legs. He refuses to go to physical therapy, remains at home on the couch most of the day, complains that he can't sleep, and just wants pain medication to control his pain. The clinic sends him to see you to assess for any other pain management techniques that might improve James' pain.

His current medications are:

- oxycontin, 240 mg three times per day
- oxycodone, 30 mg every 4 hours as needed for pain
- robaxin
- ambien
- neurontin, 300 mg three times per day

Questions to Consider

1. What adjustments would you make to the medications? Would you increase the Oxycontin dose?
2. What would you do to treat the neuropathic component of his pain?
3. Does James need an opioid treatment agreement?
4. What screening tools would you use for James?
5. Comparing the risk–benefit ratio for the medication regimen James is on, what would you suggest?
6. What guideline would you use to best treat his pain?

REFERENCES

American Academy of Pain Medicine & American Pain Society. (1997). *The use of opioids for the treatment of chronic pain.* Glenview, IL: American Pain Society.

D'Arcy, Y., & Bruckenthal, P. (2009). Elements of safe prescribing. *Journal of the Academy of Nurse Practitioners.*

Fishbain, D. A., Cole, B., Lewis, J., Rosamoff, H. L., & Rosamoff, R. S. (2008). What percentage of chronic nonmalignant pain patients exposed to chronic opioid analgesic therapy develop abuse/addicition and or aberrant drug-related behaviors? A structured evidence-based review. *Pain Medicine, 9*(4), 444–459.

Flemming, M. F., Balousek, S. L., Klessig, C. L., Mundt, M. P., & Brown, D. D. (2007). Substance use disorders in a primary care sample receiving daily opioid therapy. *Journal of Pain, 8*(7), 573–582.

Gourlay, D. L., Heit, H. A., & Almahrezi, A. (2005). Universal precautions in pain medicine: A rational approach to the treatment of chronic pain. *Pain Medicine, 6*(2), 107–112.

Passik, S., Kirsh, K. L., & Casper, D. (2008). Addiction-related assessment tools and pain management instruments for a screening, treatment planning, and monitoring compliance. *Pain Medicine, 9*(S2), S145–S166.

ADDITIONAL RESOURCES

Bruckenthal, P. (2007). Controlled substances: Principles of safe prescribing. *The Nurse Practitioner, 32*(5), 7–11.

Butler, S. F., Budman, S. H., Fernandez, K., & Jamison, R. N. (2004). Validation of a screener and opioid assessment measure for patients with chronic pain. *Pain, 112*, 65–75.

Butler, S. F., Budman, S. H., Fernandez, K. C., Houle, B., Benoit, C., Katz, N., & Jamison, R. N. (2007). Development and validation of the current opioid misuse measure. *Pain, 130*, 144–156.

Chou, R., & Huffman, L. H. (2007). Medications for acute and chronic low back pain: A review of evidence for an American Pain Society/ American College of Physicians clinical practice guideline. *Annals of Internal Medicine, 147*(7), 505–514.

D'Arcy, Y. (2007). *Pain management: Tools and techniques for nursing professionals.* Marblehead, MA: HCPro.

D'Arcy, Y., & McCarberg, B. (2007). NP prescribing authority for opioids. *PainMedicine News, 5*(1), 125–26.

International Association for the Study of Pain. (n.d.). Retrieved from www.iasp.org

IV

Treating Common
Chronic Pain Conditions

11

Low Back Pain

OVERVIEW

Low back pain (LBP) is a very common complaint. Most Americans have experienced some form of the condition at some time in their lives. Statistics indicate that it affects both men and women in equal numbers and occurs most commonly between 30 and 50 years of age. It can be caused by a variety of injuries, such as overuse and wear and tear, but some individuals just wake up in pain with no identifiable cause for their LBP. Back pain is strongly correlated with spinal disc generation and can be produced by degeneration of the lumbar zygapophysial joints (Cohen & Raja, 2007; Luoma et al., 2000). Chronic conditions, such as osteoarthritis, can also cause vertebral disc degeneration, resulting in LBP.

Sometimes, patients may feel that they did something wrong or secretly blame themselves for lifting a box that was too heavy that results in damage to their back. Because the back governs our ability to move and function, LBP that limits activities can be very distressing. The patient has to deal not only with LBP but also with wide-ranging and significant losses, such as loss of work time and loss of income. Lastly, the ongoing pain can lead to depression and added stress.

Most LBP patients will try home remedies, such as heat or analgesic balms, to self-treat the pain initially. Some individuals do well with mild analgesics and can remain active. Others have more severe pain and require more aggressive intervention. In addition, many

217

LBP patients have difficulty sleeping, adding to difficulty coping with the situation. Many ultimately feel hopeless or worthless.

In a 2002 study of 31,044 adult patients that took place over a 3-month period, 26% of the respondents reported experiencing LBP that lasted for at least a day. This equates to about one-fourth of U.S. adults reporting that they had back pain within the past 3 months. LBP is the leading patient complaint seen by physicians in the United States. In general, using data analysis that generalized the study findings, the authors concluded that about one-half of all adults have LBP in any year, and about two-thirds have at least 1 day of back pain during the past 3 months. Additionally, the authors found that approximately 15% of adults report "frequent" back pain that can last more than 2 weeks annually (Deyo, Mirza, & Martin, 2006).

There are two types of costs related to LBP and LBP management. First, there is the direct cost of treatment. Secondly, there are the hidden costs of lost work time and reduced work performance, when workers try to work but are unable to perform at their usual level because of pain. The cost of reduced work performance has been estimated at $62 billion dollars per year. LBP is the biggest cause of work-related disability, with 5% to 8% of the patients reporting pain of severe intensity (Von Korff & Saunders, 1996). For patients with chronic LBP, one in eight loses time from work. This lost time can seriously affect the patient's ability to maintain financial status and financial independence and security.

Chronic, persistent LBP affects the patient's life in every aspect. Relationships, sexual functioning, sleep, energy levels, and self-esteem all suffer when a patient has back pain that is a constant part of daily life. Helping patients with LBP to manage their pain requires a multidisciplinary approach that can produce positive outcomes for the patient and provide satisfaction for the practitioner as well.

DIFFERENCES BETWEEN ACUTE LOW BACK PAIN AND CHRONIC LOW BACK PAIN

There is a difference between acute and chronic LBP. Acute LBP is a pain that resolves within 6 to 12 weeks—no matter what treatment options are used (Hagan, Hilde, Jamtveldt, & Winnem, 2006). Treatment options for acute LBP include continued activity and the use of mild analgesics, whereas chronic LBP requires a multidisciplinary approach that includes medications and physical therapy. If the patient with acute LBP does not improve within the 12-week period, the patient is considered to have chronic LBP (Von Korff & Saunders, 1996). The percentage of patients who fall into this category is reported as 15% of the acute LBP patients (Von Korff & Saunders).

Some acute LBP occurs when patients in poor physical conditioning undertake activities that exceed their physical abilities by lifting or moving heavy objects, through overuse, or by bending or stretching in the wrong position. These individuals, sometimes labeled "weekend warriors," try to perform all the planned tasks for the weekend with little consideration as to how their bodies respond or attempt a task that simply is beyond their capability. If an individual exerts too much pressure on a vertebral disc, for example, it can herniate the disc, creating a herniated nucleus pulposus (HNP). The HNP, in turn, can create pressure on the adjacent spinal nerves, resulting in acute LBP. The HNP can require medical attention and, in more severe cases, surgical treatment. If the LBP from an HNP lasts more than 12 weeks, it becomes chronic LBP.

Other patients with LBP have conditions that predispose them to LBP. These conditions include osteoarthritis, the normal wear and tear of aging, a malignancy, and spinal stenosis, which is a narrowing of the spinal canal that occurs over time. For these patients, the pain that they experience may limit activity, impair sleep, and seriously affect their ability to maintain normal social activity. One of the goals of treatment for LBP patients is to maximize functionality and to give the patient the opportunity for the best quality of life possible.

There are some identified risk factors that predispose patients to LBP. These include:

- Poor physical condition with no regular exercise regimen
- Age older than 55 years
- Having to lift heavy loads and engage in daily hard physical labor over a period of their work lives

- Obesity
- Reduced spinal canal dimensions (spinal stenosis)
- Lower socioeconomic status and less access to health care (Dorsi & Belzberg, 2005)

As the baby boomer generation ages, it is expected that the prevalence of LBP will increase at the same time. Individuals who are at risk for LBP should be encouraged to maintain appropriate weight and to exercise regularly. Because inactivity and obesity are directly related to the occurrence of LBP, patients who are also at risk for spinal changes related to age should also be encouraged to develop and maintain a more active lifestyle to help improve their chances for better back health.

THE SPINE

The structure of the spine is really not suited to upright posture and carrying heavy body weight. Because of the way the spine is structured, it is very easy to strain or injure the back. The spine is a series of interconnected vertebrae and gelatinous discs. It is the major support structure for muscles, ligaments, and tendons of the body and serves as a protective structure for the spinal cord, which passes through the individual vertebrae in a hollowed out central ring.

The spine consists of three separate sections of vertebrae. From the top to bottom these sections are:

- Cervical: 7 vertebrae, C1-C7
- Thoracic: 12 vertebrae, T1-T12
- Lumbar: 5 vertebrae, L1-L5

Below the lumbar vertebrae is the sacrum consisting of five fused vertebrae and the coccyx with four fused vertebrae (Eathorne, 2007). LBP can occur at any level, including the sacrum. From each vertebra, a set of nerves starts at the spinal cord and exits the spine through the vertebral foramen. Depending on the level, the nerves control the various muscle groups. The area of the body that the nerves serve is called a dermatome. The dermatome schematic can be used to identify which nerve is causing the pain.

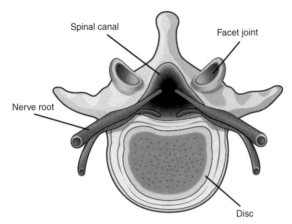

Figure 11.1 ■ Normal vertebra (cross section)

On each side of the vertebra is a wing-like projection called a transverse process that contains a small joint called a *facet joint* (Figure 11.1). These facet joints can narrow from arthritic changes, trauma, aging, or compression fractures, and nerve compression can occur. If the associated pain becomes problematic and the facet joint is the source of the pain, a steroid/local anesthetic injection can be placed directly into the joint for pain relief.

In addition to the vertebrae, each spinal process is separated by a fluid filled gelatinous disc that is composed of 60% to 70% water (Eathorne, 2007). The function of the gelatinous discs is to serve as a cushion and act as a shock absorber. These discs give height to the spine, provide for spinal mobility, and can help maintain support and posture.

A fibrous structure called an *annulus fibrosus* surrounds each disc. This wrapping consists of 12 concentric fibrous layers that help to hold the disc in place and allow the disc to absorb shock and change shape while holding the structures in place (Eathorne, 2007). As age-related or injury-related degenerative changes take place, the disc becomes less supple and compression injuries can occur—for

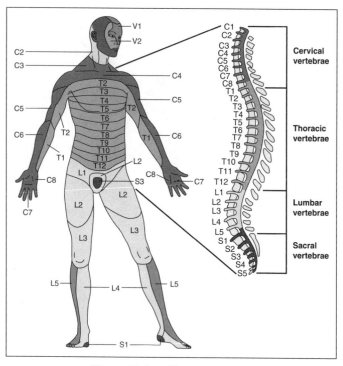

Figure 11.2 ■ Dermatome man

example, as the result of a sneeze or poor lifting technique—causing the disc to rupture through the annulus, resulting in a herniated disc. This type of injury can be particularly painful because it involves nerve root compression leading to radiculopathy, pain that radiates down one or both legs. Some treatment options, such as epidural steroid injections, have the best outcomes for patients who have a radicular component to their LBP.

The natural curvature of the spine at the cervical and lumbar area can contribute to some types of LBP (Figure 11.2). Proper posture will avoid any stress on the spinal structures. There are four normal curvatures to the spine: cervical and lumbar lordosis and thoracic and sacral kyphosis (Eathorne, 2007). Abnormal

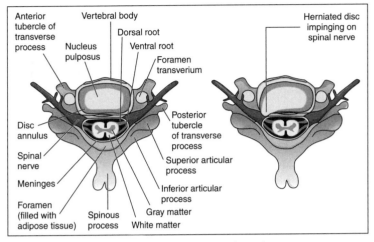

Figure 11.3 ■ Top views of vertebrae

curvatures such as *scoliosis* can cause pain related to the misalignment of the vertebra.

- Lordosis refers to the inward curve of the lumbar spine (just above the buttocks).
- Kyphosis refers to the outward curve of the thoracic spine (at the level of the ribs).
- Scoliosis is a sideways curvature of the spine and is always abnormal. (definitions from Medline Plus Medical Dictionary)

LOW BACK PAIN SYNDROME

Back pain can be classified as *axial* (focused on the low back), *referred* (pain experienced in the buttock or posterior thigh), or *radicular* (pain radiating down the leg). Aside from the common muscle strain that can cause LBP, there are several common back pain syndromes, such as HNP, facet disease, degenerative disc disease (DDD), spinal stenosis, and compression fractures (Figure 11.3). Some conditions are the result of degenerative changes, but others can be caused by trauma, poor lifting or stretching techniques, or simply a sudden sneeze.

Herniated Nucleus Pulposus

HNP as described previously is a rupture of the disc through the fibrous annulus, causing pressure on adjacent nerves. The biggest number of disc herniations is in the lumbar region (90%), with 8% in the cervical spine and 1% to 2% in the thoracic spine.

Signs and Presenting Symptoms of HPN

- Localized sudden onset of severe intensity LBP
- Radicular pain down one or both legs
- Weakened or loss of motor function, numbness in the affected extremity, or absent deep tendon reflexes
- In the cervical region, the pain may be increased with bending of the neck, turning from side to side, laughing, coughing, or straining
- Muscle spasms may occur

Diagnostic Criteria

For an HNP located in the lumbar region, diagnostic criteria includes the use of a straight leg raise, during which the back pain is reproduced when the leg is straight raised to a 90° angle. If pain is severe and there is a neurologic impairment, magnetic resonance imaging (MRI) is recommended to assist with diagnosis (Chou et al., 2007).

Treatment Options

- Medications such as acetaminophen, muscle relaxants, and opioids if the pain is severe (Chou et al., 2007)
- Lifestyle changes, such as weight loss and exercise (Chou & Huffman, 2007b)
- Perform electromyography if there is a need to identify which nerves are affected.
- Worsening of neurologic symptoms, such as a decrease in deep tendon reflexes, warrants an immediate referral for a neurosurgical or orthopedic evaluation

Degenerative Disc Disease

Because of the aging of the American population, a large number of patients will develop DDD related to the changes of aging. By age 20, the water and vascular supply to the disc decreases. By age 30, there is no vascular access to the disc, and the desiccation of the disc causes cracks; fissures begin developing in the vertebral body endplates, which is one of the causes of DDD. By age 70, 60% of the spinal discs have degenerated (Raj, 2008).

Signs and Symptoms of DDD

■ Motor weakness
■ Deep midline LBP that can radiate to buttocks or thighs
■ Sensory changes
■ Absent or diminished reflexes
■ In more severe cases, bowel or bladder dysfunction

Diagnostic Criteria

Patients with DDD may develop vertebral osteophytes (bone spurs), a condition called *spondylosis*, which can be visualized on radiographic studies and is the stiffening of the vertebrae. It can also affect the facets of the spine, and this condition is called *facet disease*. Diagnostic tests used for DDD include:

■ Provocative discography with computed tomography (CT) discography
■ Gadolinium enhanced MRI

Treatment Options

Conservative treatment with physical therapy, pain medications, gentle traction, and lifestyle changes for obese or inactive patients can be attempted. About 90% of patients can get satisfactory pain relief if the patient is willing to put in the time (Raj, 2008). Medication, surgical, and interventional treatment options include:

■ Intradiscal electrothermal therapy (IDET); see Chapter 7 on interventional pain management for more information

- Laser discectomy
- Radiofrequency ablation
- Manual percutaneous lumbar discectomy
- Endoscopic percutaneous discectomy
- Artificial disc implantation
- Glucosamine and chondroitin; similar result as IDET
- Cell-based therapies to repair degenerated cartilage (Raj, 2008)

Facet Disease

Facet disease affects approximately 15% of patients with chronic LBP. Facet disease is a common term that is applied to pain that originates in the lumbar zygapophysial joints. It is estimated that 80% of patient who report LBP and sciatica are really experiencing referred pain from facet joints (Cohen & Raja, 2007). The pain commonly called *facet syndrome* is said to be caused by a sudden rotary strain, repetitive strain, or low-grade trauma over time (Cohen & Raja, 2007).

Signs and Symptoms of Facet Disease

- LBP or buttock radiating down one or both legs, "sciatica"
- Thigh pain
- Pain along the lateral aspect of the calf

Diagnostic Criteria

- CT or MRI
- Diagnostic blocks

Treatment Options

- Conservative medication treatments include the use of acetaminophen or nonsteroidal anti-inflammatory drugs (NSAIDs); see medication information provided in Chapter 3 and in a later section in this chapter
- Conservative treatments for facet pain include exercise programs
- Yoga
- Osteopathic manipulation
- Acupuncture

■ Intra-articular steroid injections
■ Radiofrequency denervation (Cohen & Raja, 2007)

Compression Fractures

Vertebral compression fractures can occur spontaneously, especially in older patients with osteoporosis, or as the result of a lifting or bending motion. The fractures can be difficult to visualize on x-ray in the early stages but become more apparent over time. The patient will report extreme pain in the area of the fracture. One of the main causes of vertebral compression fractures is osteoporosis, which makes bones brittle and porous. It is estimated that over 100 million people worldwide and 44 million in the United States are at risk for vertebral fractures related to osteoporosis (Phillips, 2003). The consequences of these fractures results in 700,000 spinal fractures annually, with 800,000 emergency room visits, 2,600,000 outpatient visits, and the placement of 180,000 older adults in long-term care (D'Arcy, 2008).

Signs and symptoms of compression fractures include acute, localized, and constant severe pain at the site of the fracture.

Diagnostic Criteria

A standard spinal MRI will reveal the extent of the spinal compression. If medications to enhance calcium absorption are being considered, a bone density scan is required.

Treatment Options

Options for treating pain with acute compression fractures include:

■ Pain medications, such as opioids or NSAIDs if the patient can tolerate NSAIDs
■ Topical medications, such as 5% lidocaine patch
■ Bedrest
■ Braces
■ Minimally invasive techniques, such as vertebroplasty and kyphoplasty.

Vertebroplasty and kyphoplasty are techniques that use a balloon inserted through a spinal needle into the vertebra to create a space. Once the space is created a liquid cement, polymethylmethacrylate, is inserted into the space. This can reduce the amount of compression on the spinal nerve by increasing the height of the vertebra. In a systematic review of vertebroplasty and kyphoplasty, 85% of the patients with vertebroplasty and 92% of the patients with kyphoplasty reported good pain relief with the procedure (Hulme, Krebs, Fergusson, & Berlemann, 2006). Pain ratings with the use of vertebroplasty were reduced from 8.2 on a 0 to 10 pain intensity scale to 3.0, and with kyphoplasty, the pain ratings were decreased from 7.4 to 3.4 (Hulme, Krebs, Fergusson, & Berlemann, 2006).

Two other mechanical spinal conditions can cause LBP:

- *Spondololysis* is a physical defect in the vertebral arch because of mechanical stress, such as hyperextension of the spinal body. Physical complaints include constant LBP and at times motor or sensory loss.
- *Spondolisthesis* is a slipping of the vertebra, where one overrides the lower vertebra. Severe pain, radicular symptoms, and bowel and bladder dysfunction can occur, and the patient can experience weakness in the lower extremities.

PRACTICE RECOMMENDATIONS FOR DIAGNOSING AND TREATING LOW BACK PAIN FROM THE AMERICAN COLLEGE OF PHYSICIANS AND THE AMERICAN PAIN SOCIETY

Nonspecific LBP complaints account for about 85% of patients who are seen in primary care clinics (Chou et al., 2007). Patients with spinal stenosis and herniated discs account for 3% to 4% of LBP patients, cancer 0.7%, and compression fractures 4% (Chou et al., 2007). In an effort to standardize treatment options for individuals seeking pain management for LBP. The American College of Physicians (ACP) and the American Pain Society (APS) have collaborated in developing a joint guideline that provides recommendations for diagnosing and treating LBP. The guideline provides three categories for diagnosis and treatment. These categories are:

- Nonspecific LBP
- Back pain potentially associated with radiculopathy or spinal stenosis
- Back pain potentially associated with another spinal cause (Chou et al., 2007)

Interestingly, according to the guideline, a psychosocial risk factor assessment of risk factors for low back pain is more predictive of outcome of the treatment plan than the physical examination findings or the pain severity or duration (Chou et al., 2007).

LBP PRACTICE RECOMMENDATIONS

1. In order to place the patient with LBP into the correct category for diagnosis and treatment, the first guideline recommendation is to obtain a focused history and a complete physical examination of the patient. When performing a focused assessment, include assessment of the pain: intensity, frequency, location, and duration, as well as any causative factors. In addition, pay special attention to all neurologic symptoms, such as foot drop, lower extremity weakness, bowel or bladder dysfunction, or numbness. When obtaining the history from the patients, be aware of red flags that indicate a source of pain that requires a fuller workup or a specialist referral. Red flags consist of:

- Fever and chills, indicating infection or abscess
- Night pain that is highly indicative of a malignant source for the pain
- A history of cancer with possible reoccurrence, weight loss
- Recent urinary tract infection, resulting in LBP
- Intravenous drug use with resultant LBP during withdrawal or infection (Eathorne, 2007; Fishbain, Ballantyne, & Rathmell, 2010)

> *Clinical*   As part of the assessment for LBP. The straight leg raise is rec-
> *Pearl*   ommended, along with a neurologic-exam that includes great
>   toe and foot dorsiflexion, plantar dorsiflexion, and ankle re-
>   flexes. If the straight leg raise reproduces the patient's sciatic
>   pain at a 30° to 70° increase, there is a positive finding that is
>   91% sensitive but only 26% specific for diagnosing herniated
>   disc (Chou et al., 2007; Eathorne, 2007).

2. The second recommendation in the guideline clearly states that clinicians should avoid obtaining routine imaging or other radiographic diagnostic tests in patients with nonspecific LBP (Chou, 2007). This recommendation is a result of the guideline panel research review finding that MRI, CT, and plain radiography are not related to improved outcomes (Chou, 2007). Avoiding the use of imaging decreases the amount of patient radiation exposure in the lumbar and lower abdominal area of the body. This is especially important for women of childbearing years because frequent imaging can result in exposure of reproductive organs to radiation.

3. The third recommendation of the guideline also relates to when imaging should be used and what type is advised. There is a growing body of moderate quality evidence to support a strong recommendation that patients with severe or progressive neurologic deficits or with suspected serious underlying conditions identified during the history and physical examination should have diagnostic imaging and testing (Chou, 2007). In these cases, MRI is the preferred method for imaging over CT. This is because the MRI provides increased structural visualization and reduced ionizing radiation. Immediate imaging is recommended for:

- Cancer with suspected cord compression
- Vertebral infection
- Cauda equina syndrome (Chou, 2007)

When the patient has persistent LBP with/without radiculopathy or suspected spinal stenosis, MRI is preferred over CT *only* if the patient is a candidate for surgery or epidural steroid injection (Chou, 2007). Nerve conduction studies provide little benefit in the diagnostic process for LBP.

The new guidelines examine the outcomes of various diagnostic techniques. The practice recommendations reflect using imaging techniques only if they will affect the outcome of treatment. To use imaging on patients with nonspecific LBP will only increase treatment costs, increase radiation exposure, and provide no added benefit to the outcome of treatment.

APS Recommendations for Treating Low Back Pain

How should the health care provider decide which medications to use for treating LBP? In later sections of the LBP guideline developed by the APS and ACP, information on medication use and outcomes was used to determine practice recommendations for treating LBP.

The primary care health care provider is often faced with the patient who does not feel he or she has had adequate treatment for pain if there is no prescription for medication. In a recent study, 80% of primary care patients who complained of LBP were prescribed at least one medication at their initial office visit and more than one-third were prescribed two or more drugs (Chou & Huffman, 2007a). The consistent use of prescription pain medications for LBP reinforces the prevailing consumer concept that medication is always needed and will relieve LBP. Unfortunately, medication alone may not relieve LBP, and pain medications will not always be effective for the individual patients.

Because American health care consumers expect to receive a prescription for LBP, it is important to determine just which medication will produce the best outcomes with minimal side effects. There are some categories of medication, such as acetaminophen, that are recommended, whereas other categories, such as opioids, have a narrower application indicated by the pain and primary care societies

Medication Recommendations

■ *Acetaminophen*

Acetaminophen is an over-the-counter medication that is readily available in a variety of formulations. If medicine cabinets in America were surveyed, it would be found that most would include a container of acetaminophen or a medication that contains acetaminophen. Acetaminophen has low risk when taken in dosages lower than the recommended maximum dose of 4,000 mg/day for short periods. No medication is totally benign. At doses of 4,000 mg/day, there can be asymptomatic elevations of aminotransferase even in healthy adults, but the risk profile to these increases has not been clearly identified (Chou & Huffman, 2007a). The LBP guidelines recommend acetaminophen as the treatment for acute LBP, along with the recommendation to the patient to remain as physically active as possible.

■ *Nonsteroidal Anti-inflammatory Drugs*

There are two different types of NSAIDs available for treating pain: nonselective NSAIDs and COX-2 selective NSAIDs. The nonselective NSAIDs affect both COX-1 and COX-2 prostaglandin production. The sole COX-2 selective NSAID medication, celecoxib (Celebrex), is only COX-2 selective and does not affect the COX-1 prostaglandins that protect the stomach lining. Because prostaglandins are found in other organs, including the heart and the kidneys, there are risk factors for using any type of NSAID. For this reason, the primary use for NSAIDs should be for inflammatory pain. They should be used for the *shortest period at the lowest dose* to minimize any potential for adverse events (Chou et al., 2007a).

The COX-2 medication, celecoxib (Celebrex), is available by prescription only. The nonselective NSAIDs, such as ibuprofen (Motrin), are available in over-the-counter strength preparations that are available for purchase in drug stores, supermarkets, and a number of variety stores, such as Target. Because they are so widely available, there is a definite risk of toxicity when patients are buying and using these medications without the supervision of a health care provider. Both types of NSAIDs have received recommendations for use, and all have black box warnings incorporated into their packaging.

Two significant issues to consider when prescribing NSAIDs to treat LBP involve (a) correct patient selection and (b) evaluating the risk-benefit profile. Patients with long-term needs for NSAIDs are not good candidates related to the risk of increased renovascular and cardiovascular toxicity over time. Older patients with impaired kidney function, cardiac history, or recent heart surgery are not good candidates for NSAIDs treatment for pain relief related to the increased potential for toxicity, stroke or heart attack, and bleeding, respectively.

Both types of NSAIDs have the potential for increasing cardiovascular risks and renovascular events. Nonselective NSAIDs particularly have an increased risk of gastrointestinal (GI) bleeding and ulceration (Dorsi & Belzberg, 2005). Many older patients use aspirin as a prophylaxis, and adding an NSAID to drug regimens for these patients also increases the potential for GI bleeding because of the additive effect. (See Chapter 5 for additional information on NSAIDs.)

■ *Opioid Analgesics and Tramadol*

Using opioid analgesics and tramadol hydrochloride (Ultram) to treat LBP is the third recommendation of the guideline. The role of opioids for LBP is limited. The recommendation is to reserve these medications, opioids and tramadol, for patients who have tried acetaminophen or NSAIDs and found them to be ineffective. For patients who are being considered for opioid therapy, the pain should be severe and/or disabling before the opioids are used (Chou et al., 2007).

The fear of addiction with opioid use is still a concern for many health care providers. In a survey of 400 nurse practitioners who were reporting barrier to prescribing opioids, 61% reported a fear of addicting patients and 71% reported they feared regulatory oversight of their prescribing patterns (D'Arcy, 2009a). LBP patients might require opiates for long-term treatment and many prescribers are cautious or reluctant to continue to prescribe scheduled substances on a long-term basis. In the same survey of 400 nurse practitioners, the comfort level for opioid prescribing dropped dramatically from 73% to 32% when the patient in a scenario was changed from one who needed only short-term opioids to a patient who required long-term opioid therapy for LBP (D'Arcy, 2009a).

GUIDELINES FOR CHRONIC OPIOID THERAPY

Recognizing and responding to the fears that prescribers have when prescribing opioids, a new guideline for chronic opioid therapy (COT) has been developed by the APS in conjunction with the American Academy of Pain Medicine. This guideline highlights and addresses some of the problem areas that prescribers in primary care face on a daily basis. The multidisciplinary panel that developed the COT guideline lists the following recommendations for practice when COT is being considered:

- Conduct a full history and physical examination, including diagnostic testing, and an assessment for the risk of substance abuse and misuse or addiction prior to initiation of the therapy.
- Perform a risk-benefit analysis to analyze benefit to harm for moderate to severe pain and assess for function and quality of life prior to beginning opioid treatment.
- Obtain informed consent and establish a COT management plan that includes documentation of a discussion with the patient on treatment goals, expectations, potential risks, and alternatives.
- Individualize the medication dose and titration when doing a COT trial.
- Prescribe methadone carefully, with initiation and titration being carried out by clinicians familiar with its use and risks.
- Regularly reassess patients on COT and document urine screening, pain intensity ratings, functionality, progress toward identified goals, adverse events, and compliance with the prescribed regimen.
- Perform a full assessment when aberrant behaviors, dose escalations, and high dose prescriptions occur, or when opioid rotation is considered as an option.
- Place high-risk patients on COT only when monitoring parameters can be maintained and assistance from addictionologists or mental health specialists is available.
- Counsel patients who are on COT to avoid driving when impaired.
- Prescribe minimal or no opioids for pregnant patients, unless the potential benefits outweigh the risks.
- Include a multidisciplinary team for COT and include functional restoration, psychotherapeutic interventions, and other nonopioid therapies. (Chou et al., 2009; D'Arcy, 2009b).

Conforming to the recommendations in the COT and LBP guidelines will help provide positive outcomes for patients while protecting the practice of the prescribing practitioner.

RISKS OF CHRONIC OPIOID THERAPY

Risk of Opioid Addiction

Some primary care practitioners are more comfortable prescribing a medication such as tramadol hydrochloride (Ultram) because it is not a pure opioid agonist. Ultram, a synthetic mu agonist drug combined with a selective serotonin reuptake inhibitor (SSRI), was found to provide more effective pain relief than placebo in patients with chronic LBP (Chou & Huffman, 2007a).

Practitioners who are considering prescribing long-term opioids for LBP should be aware of recent research findings related to levels of addiction. Although many practitioners fear that patients who take long-term opioids will develop addiction, the actual facts support a different view. A 38-study systematic review of opioid use for treating LBP revealed that opioids commonly are prescribed for LBP and that they provide benefit for short-term use. The benefit for long-term use was less clear (Martell, O'Connor, Kerns, Becker, Morales, et al., 2007). Additional findings from this analysis indicate a high incidence of substance abuse disorder and a 24% occurrence of aberrant medication disorder (Martell, O'Connor, Kerns, Becker, Morales, et al., 2007).

Determining the true incidence of addiction in primary care patients who take long-term opioids is difficult, and more data are needed to make a definitive finding. However, there are some studies that address this question. In one study of 800 patients seen in primary care practices for chronic pain and taking opioids, the rate of addiction was roughly 4% (Flemming, Balousek, Klessig, Mundt, & Brown, 2007). In another study, the incidence of addiction in primary care patients was found to be 0.97% in opioid naïve patients and 4.37% in those patients who had used opioids previously (D'Arcy, 2009b; Fishbain, Cole, Lewis, Rosomoff, & Rosomoff, 2008).

The low rate of addiction in these studies should reassure prescribers that, although there is a risk that addiction could occur, the majority of patients are able to take opioid medications long term without becoming addicted.

Clinical Pearl	*Opioid naïve:* A patient who has not been taking opioids prior to the start of opioid therapy *Opioid tolerant or dependent:* A patient who takes opioid medications regularly (every day) Using opioids in these two groups is very different. Opioid-tolerant patients may require more medication for new pain, such as postsurgery pain. Although opioid-naïve patients require more monitoring for adverse effects at the beginning of opioid therapy (D'Arcy, 2010).

Opioid-Induced Hyperalgesia Syndrome

Opioid-induced hyperalgesia is another very real risk of COT. When this syndrome develops, patients often will say they "hurt all over," and even normal touch can cause extreme pain. The pain intensity is considered to be much higher than the pain stimulus would indicate and is thought to be unrelated to the original pain stimulus (DuPen, Shen, & Ersek, 2007). This syndrome is considered to be an atypical hyperalgesic state caused by long-term use of opioids that create pain generation in the central nervous system and no longer require nociceptive input to create the pain sensation (DuPen, Shen, & Ersek, 2007).

With all the considerations and limitations surrounding the use of opioids for chronic LBP, there still will be patients for whom this is the only option. For these patients, the prescriber should be aware of the guidelines that provide information and guidance on practice recommendations for long-term opioid use. For those patients who are having pain that requires opioids, the positive results that the use of these medications can provide, such as improved quality of life and increased functionality, should be kept in perspective.

Other Medications for Pain

Other medications can be used alone or as a coanalgesic for adding to pain relief for patients with LBP. Antidepressants, antiseizure medications, muscle relaxants, benzodiazepines, and steroids all are viable options for adjunct pain relief. Although the evidence is mixed and the systematic reviews differ in findings, there are some indications of efficacy with some of these medications, including the following medications:

- Muscle relaxants are not all similar. There is no indication for medications to treat spasticity, such as baclofen (Lioresal), which mainly is used for acute LBP, with a short-term–high side effect profile for sedation.
- Tricylic antidepressants are an option for chronic LBP. Other antidepressants, such as SSRIs, show little evidence for use currently, but because depression is common with chronic LBP, they may be used as an adjunct for treating depression.
- Systemic steroids are not indicated for treatment of LBP with or without sciatica.
- Antiseizure medications can be used to treat LBP. The only antiseizure medication recommended for use in LBP is gabapentin (Neurontin), which has the best evidence for use in patients with radiculopathy. There is insufficient evidence to support the use of other antiseizure medications for LBP at this time.
- Benzodiazepines provide similar short-term pain relief as muscle relaxants; patients who are addicts may need increased doses.
- Herbal remedies, such as devil's claw and capsaicin, have limited benefits.

Available evidence from trials are of lower quality (Chou et al., 2007; Chou & Huffman, 2007a; D'Arcy, 2009b). Many studies only include results of the use of some medicines for 1 to 6 weeks. Such short-term data are difficult to apply to the patients with chronic LBP who require long-term medication management.

NONPHARMACOLOGIC INTERVENTIONS

Any treatment plan for LBP should include the use of nonpharmacologic interventions. This does not mean that these techniques should replace the use of medication, but simply that these options should be considered as additional means of helping to relieve pain. The research in this area is very fragmented, and there are few if any high-level research studies to support many of these practices. This simply means that there is insufficient research available at this time to demonstrate efficacy for many of these techniques. The following text includes the recommendations of the LBP guideline related to nonpharmacologic therapies.

For Acute Low Back Pain: Duration Less Than Four Weeks

- Spinal manipulation by appropriately trained providers
- Superficial heat
- Exercise therapy, both supervised and at home regimens, have not proven effective for LBP in the acute phase

Subacute Low Back Pain: Duration More Than Four, but Less Than Eight Weeks

- Interdisciplinary rehabilitation that includes a physician, physical therapy, and psychological, social, and vocational intervention can be moderately effective.
- Cognitive behavioral therapy reduces absenteeism from work.

Chronic Low Back Pain: Duration More Than Eight Weeks

- Acupuncture
- Exercise therapy
- Massage therapy
- Viniyoga style yoga
- Progressive relaxation
- Spinal manipulation
- Interdisciplinary rehabilitation
- Transcutaneous electrical nerve stimulation (TENS) has inconclusive evidence to support use (Chou & Huffman, 2007; D'Arcy, 2009b; Henschke et al., 2007; Manheimer, White, Berman, Forys, & Ernst, 2005; Milne et al., 2001)

Other Interventional Practices

Although commonly used in pain clinics and other interventional practices, there is conflicting evidence related to the use of epidural or other injections for relieving LBP (Marcus, 2008). *Prolotherapy,* the injection of irritant solutions, such as pumice or glycerol, into weakened back muscles, does not have evidence to support its use alone, but when added to a comprehensive regimen of rehabilitation, the injections are more effective than control injections (Yelland, Del Mar, Pirozzo, & Schoene, 2004).

What does this mean for the patient with LBP? There has now been some research evaluation of common techniques for relieving pain in LBP patients and indicating which practices produce the best outcomes for the patient. For the acute phase, patients should stay active and use heat, and medication such as acetaminophen and NSAIDs, if the patient is a good candidate, will produce the best outcome (Chou et al., 2007). If the pain persists, adding in a rehabilitation program and relaxation will provide benefit and reduce absenteeism from work (Chou et al., 2007).

For chronic LBP pain patients, the guidelines recommend:

- Combining medications
- Using complementary techniques, such as yoga and exercise to increase flexibility in tense muscles, swimming, or water classes
- Opioids are an option if the pain is severe or disabling
- Relaxation can help reduce stress

Additional Considerations for Managing the Patient With Low Back Pain

Patient Education

Another aspect of the LBP guidelines is to educate the patients about the syndrome and to provide information on treatment options. Some key points include:

- Explain the expected course of the LBP.
- Encourage the patient to remain active.
- Provide patients with effective self-care options, such as heating pads (Chou, 2007b).

Evaluate and Manage Depression

Many patients with LBP are depressed. It is a common occurrence and should be treated aggressively to avoid serious repercussions. Concomitant depression can be almost as disabling as LBP. In a study of 416 patients using a depressions scale (CES-CD), 18.3% of patients with chronic pain scored as clearly depressed, and 57% of the chronic pain patients studied had a major depressive episode in their lifetime. Coping with LBP as well as a major depression can be overwhelming for the patient. The nurse practitioner should be aware of the high incidence of depression with chronic pain and screen patients with chronic pain for depression so that both the depression and pain can be adequately treated.

The rate of suicide in patients with chronic pain is twice the rate of patients without pain (Tang & Crane, 2006). Patients need to be informed that depression is common with chronic pain and that antidepressant therapy can help the patients cope with the continuing pain. In order to make this interaction easier, the health care provider and the patient need to have a therapeutic relationship that allows them both to share their feelings and concerns so that an effective treatment strategy can be developed. No patient should ever feel that suicide is a good option to end pain.

Exercise

Encouraging patients to stay active in the early stages of back pain is a change in paradigm. In the past, patients would often take several days of bed rest to help recover from an acute low back injury, strain, or sprain. Using yoga, massage, relaxation, stress relief, and meditation can help build coping skills that are needed to deal with LBP.

Teach Use of Pain Intensity Scale

There should also be a discussion about what pain intensity ratings mean. Select a pain intensity scale suited to the patient's self-assessment capability and teach the patient how to use it regularly and consistently.

This will assist the primary care provider in evaluating the effectiveness of pain management interventions. Do keep in mind that patients with chronic LBP often function at higher pain ratings. If the patient says they have been able to work or perform at a good physical level, the health care provider may not perceive them to be in pain. Some patients may not "look" like they are in pain, but he or she may just be trying to get through their day in the best way possible.

Other Indicators of Functionality

Although numeric pain ratings are helpful to determine if pain medication is effective, they are not meant to be the entire method for assessing pain in patients with chronic LBP. Functionality and increases in quality of life may be more important measurement for improvement. If the patient can walk further, shop independently, and attend church, these are all goals that have true meaning for maintaining the quality of life for patients with chronic pain. Continued tracking of numeric ratings may do more harm than good if pain intensities fail to improve.

Keeping an open mind about all treatment options is beneficial for patients. Encourage patients to look beyond medication management and seek opportunities to try additional types of pain relief. Medications for chronic pain should never be seen as the only option for pain relief. Using multimodal pain management will in the end produce the best outcomes for the patient and increase the potential for optimal pain relief.

To get more information on the LBP guidelines from APS, access the website at http://www.ampainsoc.org.

Sara Stone, who is a 45-year-old patient, tells you she has had LBP for about 6 weeks. She says the back pain started when she was moving and she lifted a series of heavy boxes. She has tried a variety of treatments with little effect. She lists the things that she has tried as heat and cold, analgesic balms (Icy Hot), acetaminophen, over-the-counter ibuprofen, and a pain pill from an old surgery she had several years ago. Nothing seems to work, and the pain is very intense at night when she gets into bed. She can only tolerate the lying position for several hours, and then she gets up and sleeps the rest of the night in a recliner chair. She has an appointment with a chiropractor but thought she would see her primary care provider before she went and had an adjustment.

When you examine Sara, you note that she has pain in her lumbar spine that radiates down her left leg. When you ask her to rate the pain, she says the midback pain is a nagging pain that aches and she rates it as a 5/10. When you question her about the leg pain that radiates, she describes it as a shooting pain that increases in intensity the longer she ambulates. The radicular pain is described as an 8 out of 10 when it occurs. She describes the radiating pain as intermittent, sharp, shooting, and needlelike. It keeps her from having a good night's sleep because it wakes her periodically at night.

Sara tells you she has never had pain like this before. She has no other neurologic impairment, such as foot drop or bowel or bladder incontinence. She does have a significant neuropathic component to the pain. You send Sara for an MRI, and after reading the results, you diagnose her as having a herniated disc, HNP.

Questions to Consider

1. Consider that Sara is not a surgical candidate. What are some of the best strategies to manage her pain?
2. What types of medication will be the best option for controlling Sara's pain?
3. Should you combine your medication choices to address all the components of Sara's LBP?
4. What nonpharmacologic options are good suggestions for Sara?
5. Is Sara at risk for depression? If so, what types of treatment options will work best?

REFERENCES

Chou, R., & Huffman, L. H. (2007). Medications for acute and chronic low back pain: A review of the evidence for an American Pain Society/American College of Physicians clinical practice guideline. *Annals of Internal Medicine, 147*(7), 505–514.

Chou, R., & Huffman, L. H. (2007b). Nonpharmacologic therapies for acute and chronic low back pain: A review of the evidence for an American Pain Society/American College of Physicians clinical practice guideline. *Annals of Internal Medicine, 147*(7), 492–504.

Chou, R., Fanciullo, G. J., Fine, P. G., Adler, J. A., Ballantyne, J. C., Davies, P., . . . American Pain Society-American Academy of Pain Medicine Opioids Guidelines Panel (2009). Clinical guidelines for the use of chronic opioid therapy in chronic noncancerous pain. *Journal of Pain, 10*(2), 113–130.

Chou, R., Qaseem A., Snow, V., Casey, D., Cross, J. T. Jr., Shekelle P., Owens D. K. (2007). Diagnosis and treatment of low back pain: A joint clinical practice guideline from the American College of Physicians and the American Pain Society. *Annals of Internal Medicine, 147*(7), 478–491.

Cohen, S. P., & Raja, S. N. (2007). Pathogenesis, diagnosis, and treatment of lumbar zygapophysial (facet) joint pain. *Anesthesiology, 106*, 591–614.

D'Arcy, Y. (2008). Treating the pain of osteoporotic compression fractures. *The Nurse Practitioner, 33*(12), 8–10.

D'Arcy, Y. (2009a). Be in the know about pain management. *Nurse Practitioner, 34*(4), 43–47.

D'Arcy, Y. (2009b). Using evidence based options for treating low back pain. *Nurse Practitioner.*

D'Arcy, Y. (2010). *How to manage pain in the elderly.* Indianapolis, IN: Sigma Theta Tau.

Deyo, R. A., Mirza, S. K., & Martin, B. I. (2006). Back pain prevalence and visit rates: Estimates for U.S. national surveys, 2002. *Spine, 31*(23), 2724–2727.

Dorsi, M. J., Belzberg, A. J. (2005). Low back pain. In M. S. Wallace, & P. Staats, *Pain medicine & management.* New York, NY: McGraw-Hill.

DuPen, A., Shen, D., & Ersek, M. (2007). Mechanisms of opioid-induced tolerance and hyperalgesia. *Pain Management Nursing, 8*(3),113–121.

Eathorne, S. W. (2007). *Thoracic and lumbar spine in ACSM's primary care sports Medicine,* 2nd edition. Philadelphia, PA: Lippincott Williams & Wilkins.

Fishbain, D. A., Cole, B., Lewis, J., Rosomoff, H. L., & Rosomoff, R. S. (2008). What percentage of chronic nonmalignant patients exposed to opioid analgesic therapy develop abuse, addiction, and or aberrant drug taking behaviors? A structured evidence based review. *Pain Medicine, 9*(4), 444–459.

Fishbain, S., Ballantyne, J., & Rathmell, J. (2010). *Bonica's management of pain,* 4th edition. Philadelphia, PA: Lippincott Williams & Wilkins.

Flemming, M. F., Balousek, S. L., Klessig, C. L., Mundt, M. P., & Brown, D. D. (2007). Substance use disorders in primary care sample receiving daily opioid therapy. *Journal of Pain, 8*(7), 573–582.

Hagan, K. B., Hilde, G., Jamtveldt, G., & Winnem, M. (2006). Bed rest for acute low back pain and sciatica. *Cochrane Database of Systematic Reviews,* 3.

Henschke, N., Ostelo, R. W. J. G., van Tudler, M. W., Vlaeyen, J. W. S., Morley, S., Assendelft, W. J. J., & Main, C. J. (2007). Behavioral treatment for chronic pain. *The Cochrane Database of Sytematic Reviews,* (1), CD002014.

Hulme, P. A., Krebs, J., Fergusson, S. J., & Berlemann, U. (2006). Vertebroplasty and kyphoplasty: A systematic review of 69 clinical studies. *Spine, 31*(17), 1983–2001.

Luoma, K., Riihimaki, H., Luukkonen, R., Raininko, R., Viikari-Juntura, E. Lanninen A. (2000) Low back pain in relation to lumbar disc degeneration. *Spine, 25,* 487–492.

Manheimer, E., White, A., Berman, B., Forys, K., & Ernst, E. (2005). Meta-analysis: Acupuncture for low back pain. *Annals of Internal Medicine, 142*(8), 651–663.

Marcus, A. (2008). APS guidelines for low back pain show little love for interventional therapies. *Pain Medicine News, 6*(6).

Martell, B. A., O'Connor, P. G., Kerns, R. D., Becker, W. C., Morales, K. H., Kosten, T. R., & Fiellen, D. A. (2007). Systematic review: Opioid treatment for chronic back pain: Prevalence, efficacy, and association with addiction. *Annals of Internal Medicine, 146*(2), 116–127.

Milne S., Welch, V., Brosseau, L., Saginur, M., Shea, B., Tugwell, P., & Wells, G. (2001). Transcutaneous electrical nerve stimulation (TENS) for chronic low back pain. *Cochrane Database of Systematic Reviews,* (2), CD003008.

Phillips, F. M. (2003). Minimally invasive treatments of osteoporotic vertebral compression fractures. *Spine, 28*(15S), S45–S53.

Raj, P. P. (2008). Intervertebral disc:Anatomy-physiology-pathophysiology-treatment. *Pain Practice, 8*(1),18–44.

Tang, N. K., & Crane, C. (2006). Suicidality in chronic pain: A review of prevalence, risk factors, and psychological links. *Psychological Medicine, 36*(5), 575–586.

Von Korff, M., & Saunders, K. (1996). The course of back pain in primary care. *Spine, 21,* 2833–2837.

Yelland, M., Del Mar, C., Pirozzo, S., & Schoene, M. L. (2004). Prolotherapy injections for chronic low back pain: A systematic review. *Spine, 29*(19), 2126–2133.

ADDITIONAL RESOURCES

D'Arcy, Y. (2006). Low back pain relief. *The Nurse Practitioner, 31*(4), 17–25.

D'Arcy, Y. (2007). *Pain management: Evidence-based tools and techniques for nursing professionals.* Marblehead, MA: HCPro.

Lamminen, A. (2000). Low back pain in relation to lumbar disc degeneration. *Spine, 25,* 487–492.

12

Rheumatoid Arthritis and Osteoarthritis

OVERVIEW

Arthritis is one of the most common types of pain complaints that a primary care practitioner will see. Arthritis, along with low back pain, contributes significantly to the high number of patient visits to health care providers for patients with pain complaints. Rheumatoid arthritis (RA) and osteoarthritis (OA) are two of the most common conditions classed as arthralgias, which also includes gout, fibromyalgia, systemic lupus erythematosus (SLE), scleroderma, infectious arthritis, and bursitis.

OA alone affects more than 20 million people in the United States (American Pain Society [APS] 2002; Danter, 2009; Hitti, 2007). The estimate of costs for the osteoarthritis itself, including treatment, lost worker productivity, and physical and occupational therapy needs, is estimated at 128 billion in 2003 (Danter, 2009). By 2030, arthritis is projected to affect 20% of the population, or 67 million adults (Hootman & Helmick, 2006). As baby boomers age, it can be anticipated that the overall costs will increase dramatically.

On the other hand, RA is considered to be inflammatory arthritis (Gardner, 2010). It is one of several different diseases that are chronic and is characterized by diffuse inflammation and degeneration of the connective tissues, often characterized by joint stiffness in the morning that lasts at least 30 minutes, but it can range to several hours (Gardner, 2010). Pain improves with activity as fluid accumulated in the joints during inactivity is forced back into the system through the lymphatics.

RA is considered to be an autoimmune disease that causes degeneration of the smaller joints of the hands and feet and the larger joints of the shoulder, elbows, and knees. RA affects 2.5 million Americans (APS, 2002). RA affects about 0.5% to 1% of the world population, with a female-to-male ratio between 2:1 and 4:1 (Firestein, 2005). It is not a condition specifically of age, but it has a peak incidence between 20 and 50 years of age (APS, 2002). The complaints that bring the patient into a primary care office include fatigue, weakness, weight loss, low-grade fever, and pain in the distal joints of the hands and feet, causing difficulty and pain with normal daily tasks, such as opening jar lids or shaking hands (Gardner, 2010).

The pain of both of these conditions can be severe and limiting. Some patients describe the pain as deep aching. For OA, the pain from joint degeneration and cartilage loss will often be described as aching with bone grating, or *crepitus*, which is audible when the joints flex and extend. It is also important to consider that patients with arthritis in general can have both chronic baseline pain and flares of acute pain when exacerbation of the disease occurs. For RA, it is important to treat the condition early and intervene with treatment that will control the pain and decrease the amount of joint destruction. Although both conditions affect bones, the cause and treatment options are different, but pain control is an important element in treating both conditions.

Clinical Pearl	Diagnosing OA can be done through a history of pain and x-rays showing a narrowing of joint space. RA is diagnosed by a history of polyarthritis for 3 months and inflammation of the joints (Danter, 2009).
	If the diagnosis of arthritis is being considered, examining synovial fluid can provide some additional information. For RA, look for cloudy fluid, with a reduced viscosity caused by the breakdown of hyaluronate and the formation of a fibrin clot. There will also be an elevated cell count consisting of mainly neutrophils ranging from 5,000–25,000 cells per cubic millimeter (Gardner, 2010).

OSTEOARTHRITIS

OA is defined as a degenerative joint disease characterized by the destruction of articular cartilage and overgrowth of bones. It is considered a disease of aging. Most older adults will have some element of the condition. The natural progression of the disease is the result of cartilage loss in weight-bearing joints, such as knees and hips, which in turn cause mechanical changes, a localized tissue response, and a decrease in function (APS, 2002). Although the older patient is the most common sufferer, there is a small group of individuals who are younger and may develop OA through repetitive stress on joints or from a trauma resulting in joint injury (APS, 2002). OA of the knee is more common in women, and OA of the hip is more common in men, 55 years of age and older (Acheson & Collart, 1975).

There are three classifications of osteoarthritis:

- Localized: involves Heberden's nodes, which are nodes located on the joints of the fingers, and no other joint involvement
- Generalized: involves three or more joints or joint groups, flares, Heberden's nodes, and a familial pattern
- Erosive: primarily affects hands; 15% of patients also have RA

Causes of osteoarthritis include the following:

- Trauma
- Congenital disorders (e.g., hip dysplasia)
- Neuropathic joint disease
- Inflammatory disorders
- Bleeding disorders
- Corticosteroid injections
- Gout
- Cushing's disease or acromegaly
- Obesity
- Muscle weakness

The joints that OA commonly affects include the following:

- Knees
- Hips
- Feet
- Ankles
- Cervical and lower spine
- Distal interphalangeal joints
- Proximal interphalangeal joints (APS, 2002)

For patients with OA, the pain can be very limiting. Because rest tends to reduce the intensity of the pain, many patients tend to adopt a more sedentary lifestyle. This type of inactivity leads to deconditioning and loss of muscle strength and mass. In reality, activity is essential for maintaining joint health and keeping muscles strong enough to support daily activity. Many OA patients report a feeling of morning stiffness or stiffness that can occur with prolonged sitting. This stiffness will resolve when activity is performed, but pain may limit the ability of the patient to keep active. The stiffness while sitting is called a "gel" phenomenon—that is, a period of stiffness that resolves in approximately 20–30 minutes (APS, 2002). Patients may need to consider using an analgesic medication to help control pain when activity is being performed or if sitting for longer periods.

If patients do not remain active, the cycle of pain, inactivity, and deconditioning will continue, with the loss of function and disability increasing. Resultant weakening of the quadriceps muscles and malalignment of the knee can create mechanical injury to the medial or lateral side of the knee, increasing weakness and pain, and negatively affect functionality. Patients with hip OA can have night pain in the hip, affecting sleep (Gardner, 2010).

Diagnosing a patient with OA includes the use of radiographic studies to examine the joint spaces. Laboratory values may have normal values. On aspiration, the synovial fluid of OA patients will be straw colored, have good viscosity, and have low cell counts (less than 2,000 white cells) (Gardner, 2010).

All patients with chronic pain have the potential for developing depression. For patients with OA, the social isolation and loss of ability to function can have profound effects. Because this condition mainly affects older patients, the loss of simple pleasures, such as gardening, church attendance, or even shopping for household needs, can be depressing. Coupled with the pain and social isolation that OA can cause, the situation can seem to be personally diminishing. The patient may feel a loss of self-esteem and worth.

Because older patients with OA may have many comorbidities, screening for depression may not be addressed, or the patients may deny that they are depressed. Recommendations from a study of 1,800 depressed older adults found the following:

- Pain and depression screening should be performed for all patients with a chronic illness and those who have symtomatic OA.
- Treating depression, when combined with patient education on self management was an effective therapy.
- Using a multimodal approach to treating pain and depression can improve treatment outcomes.

Because OA is common and affects mainly older patients, assessing the patient for pain and functionality can be integral to making changes in treatment that can provide a higher quality of life for these patients. Encouraging an older patient in pain who may not see or understand the benefit of regular movement and exercise can be a tough situation for the health care provider. Using the best treatment options can help the older patient move easier and increase the potential for maintaining functionality at the highest level.

Treatment Options for Osteroarthritis

Treating the pain of OA is key to retaining quality of life, managing pain, and maintaining functionality, and in lessening comorbidities such as depression. Recommendations for treating OA pain include the following:

- acetaminophen
- Nonsteroidal anti-inflammatory drugs (NSAIDs), oral or topical, and COX2 medications only for patients who are good candidates and with caution in some highly selected individuals

- Weight reduction
- Physical therapy
- Intra-articular injections, with steroids or injectable solutions for joint lubricating, such as sodium hyaluronate or hylan G-F 20
- Lidocaine patch over painful area
- Topical analgesic balms, such as capsaicin
- Physical therapy, transcutaneous electrical nerve stimulation (TENS) units, iontophoresis, pool-based physical therapy programs (balineotherapy), assistive devices such as a cane
- Arthritis self-management program
- Joint replacements (American Geriatrics Society, 2002; APS, 2002, 2005)

The Osteoarthritis Research Society International (OARSI) Guidelines, 2007 and 2008, also provide some direction for selecting appropriate medication and interventional options. The focus of these guidelines was to:

- Reduce joint pain and stiffness
- Maintain and improve joint mobility
- Reduce physical disability and handicap
- Improve health-related quality of life
- Limit progression of joint damage
- Educate patients about OA and management (Zhang et al., 2008)

The OARSI Guidelines also recommend both nonpharmacologic and pharmacologic interventions. OARSI pharmacologic recommendations include the following:

- Acetaminophen as first-line treatment: limit to 4 grams per day and reduce amount in patients with hepatic or renal disease or alcoholic patients.
- NSAIDs provide better relief than acetaminophen but have significant, life-threatening, serious adverse effects. Long-term use should be avoided. See information in Section 2, Chapter 3 on risk benefits of NSAID use.
- Topical medications, such as capsaicin, and topical NSAIDs, such as diclofenac, may also have risk-benefit recommendations related to side effect profile.
- Trial opioid therapy when other agents are ineffective or contraindicated. The American Geriatrics Society endorses the use of opioids in

older patients when severe pain, pain-related functional impairments, or decreased quality of life is due to pain (see Section 2, Chapter 4 for choices of opioids).

- Glucosamine or chondroitin sulfate may provide some symptomatic relief.
- Intra-articular injections may provide relief.

OARSI nonpharmacologic recommendations include the following:

- Patient education on osteoarthritis and self-management
- Physical therapy to decrease pain and improve function
- Aerobic activity to maintain muscle strength, such as water aerobics
- Weight loss
- Regular telephone contact
- Additional modalities, such as canes, braces, shoe inserts, TENS units, and acupuncture, and thermal techniques, such as heat and ice

When all of these interventions, medications, and interventional options fail, surgery is the final consideration. There are many patients who choose a total joint replacement as an option for reducing pain and increasing functionality.

OARSI recommends the following surgeries as options for patients with osteoarthritis:

- Total knee or hip replacement
- Unicompartmental knee replacement
- Osteotomy and joint preserving procedures
- Joint lavage and arthroscopic debridement
- Joint fusion when joint replacement fails

No matter which therapeutic option a patient with OA chooses, the relationship with the health care provider is paramount to the success of the intervention. Losing weight and exercising may be a big undertaking for the patient with OA, but positive reinforcement from the health care provider and use of techniques, such as water exercises or water aerobics, can help the patient get a start on a difficult process. Being sensitive to the patient's pain and using a variety of multimodal pain relief options will also make the entire process more tolerable to the patient. Measuring patient outcomes and showing improvement in function will help patients understand the benefit of the treatment plan.

RHEUMATOID ARTHRITIS

RA has a different cause than OA. It is considered to be one of the autoimmune diseases with the joint damage primarily found in the synovial tissue (APS, 2002; Danter, 2009). There have been many theories as to the cause of the disease, including Epstein-Barr virus or mycobacterial infection and environmental factors (APS, 2002).

The criteria for diagnosing RA include:

- Persistent symmetrical polyarthritis for more than 3 months, involving the small joints in the hands and feet
- Presence of persistent systematic symptoms, such as fatigue, anemia, and weight loss
- Presence of rheumatoid nodules
- Exclusion of other causes of autoimmune systemic disorders, such as SLE
- Elevated erythrocyte sedimentation rate (ESR)
- Normocytic-normochromic anemia
- Positive rheumatoid factor (RF) in 80% of the patients
- Cyclic citrullinated peptide: 75% sensitive and 96% specific for RA
- Radiographic studies in the early phase will show only articular osteopenia and soft-tissue swelling. Later studies can find similar findings as in OA, joint space narrowing, and erosion of the joint margins.

RA has a large number of systematic effects that are not present in OA patients. These include chronic synovitis, with erosion of the tendons, ligaments, and cartilage (Danter, 2009). Carpal tunnel syndrome is a common occurrence. Other organs may be affected as well. There is an increased risk of cardiovascular disease related to the ongoing inflammatory process (Danter, 2009), and lungs may develop RA lung disease, vasculitis, or Sjogren's disease (Strand, Scudder, & Fosam, 2009).

Patients who have a poorer prognosis with RA include the following:

- Patients with limitation in function
- Extra-articular manifestations (e.g., vasculitis)
- RF positivity
- Elevated c-reactive protein and/or ESR
- Older age
- Female gender
- Genotype (HLA-DRB1)
- Possibly cigarette smoking (Strand, Scudder, & Fosam, 2009)

Treatment Options for Rheumatoid Arthritis

The treatment plan for RA is focused on controlling pain and limiting joint destruction. Patients with early signs of aggressive disease are treated with a more complex combination therapy early in the disease to deter joint destruction, control pain, and inhibit decreased functionality. The tried and true treatment plan is based on a pyramid, starting with the following:

- Again, caution is advised for NSAIDs (see section in Section 2, Chapter 3 on risks and benefits of NSAIDs combined with education, physical, and occupation therapy).
- Adding disease-modifying antirheumatic drugs (DMARDs) early in the disease increases medication-induced disease remission rates by 50% when combined with methotrexate and anti–tumor necrosis factor (anti-TNF) biologics (Gardner, 2010).
- Biologic agents, such as etanercept, infliximab, and adalimumab
- Glucocorticosteroids (Strand, Scudder, & Fosam, 2009)

For symptom control, NSAIDs and steroids may be useful; for halting joint destruction, a DMARD is indicated. The recommended DMARDs include the following:

- Methotrexate, which is used in combination with another medication that seems to provide better effect. Onset of action is 3–8 weeks.
- Hydroxychloroquine is used for early to mild synovitis. It takes 8–12 weeks to become effective.

- Minocycline is less commonly used.
- Sulfasalazine is used for less severe disease. Onset of effect is 4 to 8 weeks (Gardner, 2010; Table 12.1).

Biologic agents are the newest addition to the drugs that can be used to decrease the inflammatory response. These agents, such as TNF, are effective for improving physical function, improving disease activity, increasing quality of life, and showing radiographic improvement in joint destruction[1] (Strand, Scudder, & Fosam, 2009). The American College of Rheumatology (ACR) recommendations for biologic agents for treating RA include the following:

- etanercept
- infliximab
- adalimumab
- abatacept
- rituximab

For patients with active disease that does not respond to single therapy, a combination of a DMARD and a biologic is often prescribed, and the outcomes are better than with a single agent alone (Gardner, 2010; Strand, Scudder, & Fosam, 2009). As a bridge agent, glucocorticoid 5 to 10 mg per day can be given until the DMARD action starts (Gardner, 2010). Because these medications can be toxic, before starting DMARD therapy, the ACR recommends a complete blood count, liver transaminase level, and serum creatinine level. Additionally, the ACR recommends hepatitis B and C testing, routine tuberculosis screening, and an ophthalmologic exam for retinopathy (Strand, Scudder, & Fosam, 2009). Patients should also be cautioned about pregnancy given the toxic nature of the medications and the patients will need education about birth control usage. Because these medications may induce immunosuppression, routine vaccinations for chronic disease should be given, but some live vaccines should be avoided with methotrexate, leflunomide, and all biologic agents (Strand, Scudder, & Fosam,

---

[1] This may not be effective in 30% to 40% of patients (Strand, Scudder, & Fosam, 2009).

Table 12.1 ■ *Dosing Recommendations for DMARDs*

Drug	Dose Range	Route	Serious Side Effects	Monitoring
hydroxychloroquine	200–600 mg/day	PO	Renal toxicity, neuromyopathy	Q 6–12 mos funduscopic and visual field exam
sulfasalazine	1,000–3,000 mg/day	PO	Leukopenia, sulfa hypersensitivity	CBC, platelets q 2–4 wk for 3 mos then CBC q 3 mos
methotrexate	7.5–25 mg/wk	PO, IM, SQ	Bone marrow suppression, pneumonitis, hepatoxicity	CBC, platelets, aspartate aminotransferase, albumin, and albumin q 4–8 wks
leflunomide	10–20 mg/day after 100 mg/day for 3 days as a loading dose	PO	Hepatoxicity, GI distress, diarrhea, alopecia	LFTs q mo for 6 mos then every 3 mos. CBC early in course of treatment
etanercept	25 mg twice per week to 50 mg once a week	IM, SQ	Local injection site reaction, increased risk of infections, leukopenia, severe hepatitis in hepatitis B carriers, multiple sclerosis–type illness	Baseline CBC, LFT, hepatitis B, PPD; CBC, LFTs every 3–6 mos
infliximab	Initial dose 3 mg/kg 2 wk: 5 mg/kg; 6 wk: 5 mg/kg; q 4–8 wk 5–10 mg/kg	IV	Reactivation of TB, leukopenia, increased risk of infection, SLE-like disease, tumor risk uncertain, infusion reactions	Baseline CBC, LFT, hepatitis B, PPD; CBC, LFTs every 3–6 mos
adalimumab	40 mg	SQ	Similar to infliximab	Baseline CBC, LFT, hepatitis B, PPD; CBC, LFTs every 3–6 mos

Abbreviations: CBC, complete blood count; GI, gastrointestinal; IM, intramuscularly; IV, intravenously; LFT, liver function test; PO, by mouth; PPD, purified protein derivative; q, every; SLE, systemic lupus erythematosus; SQ, subcutaneously; TB, tuberculosis.
Source: Adapted from Gardner, 2010.

2009). Additional supplements, such as calcium 1,000–1,500 mg/ day and 400 units of vitamin D, should be given to patients on daily steroids to decrease inflammatory effect (Gardner, 2010).

The inflammation, pain, and activity limitations of RA can be devastating to patients. Because some of the patients are younger, their ability to work can be adversely affected. Compliance with the medication regimen is extremely important for the patient, and the health care provider will need to assess the patient routinely for compliance and any adverse effects that are limiting full compliance with the medications.

Because the patient with RA may be anemic, anorexic, or losing weight, it is important to discuss nutrition with the patients. Using a diet history can provide insight into the patient's usual eating pattern. Small frequent meals may be needed for anorexic patients, and supplementation for vitamin D, calcium, high protein, and iron may be needed (Danter, 2009).

Other nonpharmacologic therapies can also be beneficial. Activity and exercise are essential for maintaining good weight and joint mobility. Hydrotherapy or water exercise can help reduce the weight on the joint while moving during the exercises. Simple walking is also an excellent form of exercise with low physical impact.

Acupuncture is used for treating many chronic pain conditions. RA studies have shown that it is only effective when used in conjunction with medications; for OA, acupuncture has only been studied in knee and hip patients. Other therapies to consider for RA include ice and topical capsaicin creams (Danter, 2009).

SUMMARY

There is no known cure for either OA or RA. That means that the focus of treatment is to control pain, maximize functionality, retain the current state of joint health, and help the patient learn to cope with chronic illness. Maintaining a good patient–provider relationship can help the patient accept the needed therapies and comply with treatment regimens.

Cindy Jones is a 35-year-old office worker. She has been complaining of pain in her hands for some time, and she feels fatigued but has considered that this is related to the needs of her two grammar school aged children and her job. She feels cold frequently and seems to have very little energy. She has been calling into work as ill at least three times per month for the past 6 months on a regular basis. Her boss speaks to Cindy and says she should see her health care provider to get a better idea of what is making her ill. She tells Cindy that the regular absences are making it difficult on her coworkers because they have to cover Cindy's responsibilities when she is gone. Cindy agrees to see her health care provider.

When Cindy sees her health care provider, she tells him, "I just feel so tired all the time, and my hands just ache. I have tried a bunch of topical creams and some over-the-counter medication like acetaminophen and naproxen, but nothing really seems to make it better. I keep having to call in sick, and my boss is getting concerned about my absences. I have to support my two little girls, and I just don't know what I'll do if I lose my job." When you question Cindy about other sites for pain, she indicates she has been having some pain in her feet as well, and her shoes often feel tight.

Lab results on Cindy show a positive RF and elevated ESR. A physical exam of Cindy's hands reveals rheumatoid nodules on the finger joints and warmth and swelling in the hand joints. There is some fluid accumulation at each of the joints in her fingers. You diagnose Cindy with RA.

Questions to Consider

1. What are the differences between the patient presentation with RA and OA?

2. What type of medication would be of benefit to Cindy?

3. If Cindy is willing to try some nonpharmacologic interventions, which one would you suggest?

4. Given Cindy's age, should you be concerned about her lungs, heart, or other organ systems. Why or why not?

5. What other types of effects from RA should you be assessing?

REFERENCES

Acheson, R. M., & Collart, A. B. (1975). New Haven survey of joint diseases. XVII. Relationship between some systemic characteristics and osteoarthrosis in a general population. *Annals of the Rheumatic Diseases*, *34*, 379–387.

American Geriatrics Society. (2002). The management of persistent pain in older persons. *Journal of the American Geriatrics Society*, *50*:S205–S224.

American Pain Society. (2002). *Guideline for the management of pain in osteoarthritis, rheumatoid arthritis and juvenile chronic arthritis.* Glenview, IL: American Pain Society.

American Pain Society. (2005). *Pain control in the primary care setting.* Glenview IL: The Society.

Danter, J. H. (2009). Alleviating the pain of arthralgias. *The Nurse Practitioner*, *34*(9), 40–46.

Firestein, G. S. (2005). Etiology and pathogenesis of rheumatoid arthritis. In E. D. Harris, Jr., R. C. Budd, M. C. Genovese, et al. (Eds.). *Kelley's textbook of rheumatology* (7th ed.). Philadelphia, PA: Saunders.

Gardner, G. C. (2010). Painful neuropathies. In S. M. Fishman, J. C. Ballantyne, & J. P. Rathmell (Eds.), *Bonica's management of pain* (4th ed.). Philadelphia, PA: Lippincott Williams and Wilkins.

Hitti, M. (2007). *As boomers age, arthritis costs rise.* Retrieved from http://arthritis.webmd.com/news/20070427/as-boomers-age-arthritis-costs-rise

Hootman, J. M., & Helmick, C. G. (2006). Projections of US prevalence of arthritis and associated activity limitations. *Arthritis & Rheumatism, 54*, 226–229.

Strand, V., Scudder, L., & Fosam, H. (2009). *Rheumatoid arthritis: Treatment selections for the complex patient.* Retrieved from http://www.cme.medscape.com

Zhang, W., Moskowitz, R. W., Nuki, G., Abramson, S., Altman, R. D., Arden, N., . . . Tugwell, P. (2008). OARSI recommendations for the management of hip and knee osteoarthritis, Part II: OARSI evidence-based, expert consensus guidelines. *Osteoarthritis and Cartilage, 16*, 137–162.

ADDITIONAL RESOURCES

American Academy of Orthopedic Surgeons (AAOS). (2008). *AAOS guideline for the treatment of osteoarthritis of the knee (non-arthroplasty).* Retrieved from www.guideline.gov

Brandt, K. (2003). *Diagnosis and nonsurgical management of osteoarthritis* (third edition). Professional Communications Inc. Caddo, OK: CDC. Arthritis. Retrieved from http://www.cdc.gov/arthritis/data

Budd, R. C., Genovese, M. C., et al. (Eds.). *Kelly's textbook of rheumatology* (7th ed.). Philadelphia: Saunders.

Saag, K. G., Teng, G. G., Patkar, N. M., Anuntiyo, J., Finney, C., Curtis, J. R., et al. (2008). American College of Rheumatology 2008 recommendations for the uses of nonbiologic and biologic disease-modifying antirheumatic drugs in rheumatoid arthritis. *Arthritis & Rheumatism, 59*, 762–784.

13

Fibromyalgia

OVERVIEW

Fibromyalgia, is it a real disease or not? The fibromyalgia debate has been going on for many years. For some practitioners, the syndrome is believed to be psychological in origin, but many patients who suffer from fibromyalgia can tell you that it definitely is not something they are imagining. It is a real illness that can strike without warning, cause significant pain and suffering, and negatively affect quality of life.

Fibromyalgia may start out as achy feelings at certain points in the body, the hips or shoulders, for example. The pain seems to change location, and a generalized aching, sleep disturbance, or extreme fatigue can be the problem that drives the patient to see a health care provider. Because the pain complaints are so vague and affect different areas of the patient's life, it is very difficult to pin down the source of the problem until the patient has been seen repeatedly over a period of time, perhaps years.

What also makes the diagnosis difficult is the variation in the symptoms. Sometimes the pain is better, at other times it can be debilitating. The changes in symptomatology and intensity make it hard for the health care provider to develop a comprehensive plan of care to deal with the pain, fatigue, memory lapses, and sleep disturbances. There is also wide variation in the degree of disability with the condition between patients. These differences in patients and symptoms add to the confusion about what fibromyalgia is and is not.

263

Fibromyalgia Syndrome

Fibromyalgia syndrome (FMS) affects 2% to 5% of the general patient population in the United States. However, the syndrome is more prevalent in women, 3.5% to 7%, than in men, 0.5% to 2% (Hadhazy et al., 2007). In older women, the prevalence of FMS increases to 7% (Hadhazy et al., 2007). Because of the higher prevalence in women, FMS has been relegated to the more minor conditions and minimized as a health care problem. More recent research has demonstrated some direct causal factors that point to a central nervous system neuropathic origin for the pain and have made health care providers more confident in diagnosing and treating the condition.

Patients who are diagnosed with FMS should have the major complaint of widespread axial pain above and below the waist at 11 of 18 tender points for more than 3 months (Wolfe et al., 1990). These tender points are in specific locations that include the trapezius, low-cervical area, and gluteal and lateral epicondyle (Figure 13.1).

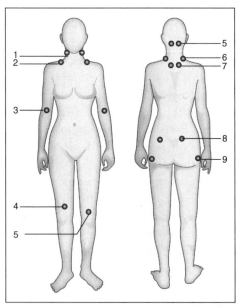

Figure 13.1 ■ Tender points

Clinical Pearl — To perform a tender point assessment, palpate the tender point by pressing each point for 4 seconds at 1 kg per second until 4 kg is achieved (Wolfe et al., 1990). The point should be depressed using the thumb until the nail becomes whitened from the pressure (Exhibit 13.1A & B).

Exhibit 13.1A

Tender Points Survey

Assessing the presence of widespread pain

Directions for physicians: Present the following figures to your patients. Ask them to fill in the areas where they have felt pain for 3 months or longer.

Directions for patients: On the figures below, color in all areas where you have experienced pain for 3 months or longer.

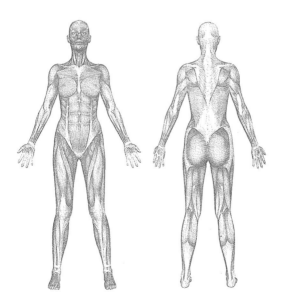

Copyright © Pfizer Inc. Reproduced with permission.

Exhibit 13.1B

Performing the Manual Tender Point Survey
Scoring sheet

Instructions for patient

Give the patient the following instructions:
"Various areas of your body will be examined for pain. Please say 'Yes' or 'No' to indicate whether there is any pain when I press a specific point."

If a patient responds, "Yes" to indicate a site is painful, the examiner should assess the patient's perception of the pain severity by asking her/him to rate the pain on a 0 to 10 scale.

In addition, explain the pain rating scale to the patient:
"I want you to rate the intensity of the pain on a scale from 0 to 10, where 0 is no pain and 10 is the worst pain that you have ever experienced."

Directions: After palpating each tender point, ask the patient to asses the amount of pain on a scale of 0 to 10 (0 = no pain; 10 = worst pain). Record the patient's response below.

SEATED position	Right	Left
Mid-forehead (control point)	1. ____	
Occiput: Suboccipital muscle insertions	2. ____	3. ____
Trapezius: Midpoint of upper border	4. ____	5. ____
Supraspinatus: Above medial border of scapular spine	6. ____	7. ____
Gluteal: Upper outer quadrant of buttocks	8. ____	9. ____
Low cervical: Anterior aspect of intertransverse space of C5–7	10. ____	11. ____
Second rib: Second costochondral junction	12. ____	13. ____
Lateral epicondyle: 2 cm distal to epicondyle	14. ____	15. ____
Right forearm (control point): junction of proximal $^{2}/_{3}$ & distal $^{1}/_{3}$	16. ____	
Left thumbnail (control point)	17. ____	
SIDE position		
Greater trochanter: Posterior to trochanteric prominence	18. ____	19. ____
SUPINE position		
Knee: Medial fat pad proximal to the joint line	20. ____	21. ____

Number of positive tender points (those with a score of 2 or greater) ____

Note that tender points 1, 16 and 17 are control points and do not count toward the total number of positive tender points.

Source: Okifujl A, Turk DC, Sinclair JD, Starz TW, Marcus DA. A standardized manual tender point survey. I. Development and determination of a threshold point for the identification of positive tender points in fibromyalgia syndrome. *Journal of Rheumatology* 1997;24(2):377–383.

Additional complaints can include the following:

- Fatigue
- Morning stiffness
- Altered sleep patterns
- Mood disturbances—20% to 40% at diagnosis; lifetime, 70%
- Cognitive loss
- Irritable bowel/bladder
- Restless legs
- Headaches
- Temporomandibular joint pain
- Anxiety
- Depression
- Panic attacks (American Pain Society [APS], 2005; D'Arcy & McCarberg, 2005; Rao et al., 2008; Wolfe et al., 1990)

New diagnostic criteria are being reviewed by the American College of Rheumatology that incorporate the use of a patient questionnaire that can be used to derive a symptom severity index to augment the use of the tender point examination. Given the wide variety of presentations of FMS and the skepticism of some health care providers about the condition, the patient who is diagnosed with FMS generally has been through a long period of uncertainty and numerous tests to rule out other conditions, such as rheumatoid arthritis or lupus. Because there is no test that can definitively prove a diagnosis of FMS, the negative results of all the testing can erode the patient's confidence. These patients require an empathic approach to get the full benefit of treatment and interventions.

Other diagnoses to exclude are:

- Rheumatoid arthritis
- Systemic lupus erythematosus
- Osteoarthritis
- Ankylosing spondylitis
- Lyme disease
- Epstein-Barr virus (EBV)
- Other soft-tissue disorders, such as myofascial pain
- Hypothyroidism
- Spinal stenosis
- Cervical myelopathy
- Major depressive disorder
- Use of statins (HMG-CoA reductase inhibitors)

It may take as long as 5 years for a patient to get a diagnosis of FMS. To get the diagnosis, the patient with fibromyalgia seeks help from a number of practitioners. Forty-six percent of the patients consult between 3 and 6 health care providers, whereas 25% see more than 6 consultants.

New Ideas in the Pathophysiology of Fibromyalgia

Originally, fibromyalgia was thought to be a condition associated with the EBV, Lyme disease, and other inflammatory diseases, but no definitive links have been established. There was also a consideration that fibromyalgia could be divided into a primary condition that occurred with no precipitating event and secondary fibromyalgia that was thought to be associated with stress, emotional distress, viral infection, or surgery (D'Arcy & McCarberg, 2005). Current research is finding evidence that the widespread pain of fibromyalgia may be a form of centrally mediated neuropathic pain. The term *central amplification* of the pain response is being used to account for the highly sensitized pain response that patients with fibromyalgia experience. This can be exemplified by patients who cannot tolerate the pressure, and subsequent pain, of a hug.

Fibromyalgia pain is not just a series of nociceptive stimuli activating the ascending neural pain pathway; it also includes the descending neural pathways and inhibitory mechanisms for pain. The patient with fibromyalgia may report exquisitely tender point pain that is very similar to allodynia. This augmentation of response is connected to the development of wind-up produced in the dorsal horn neurons as a result of activation of N-methyl-D-aspartate (NMDA) and NK1 receptors (Rao et al., 2008). NMDA receptors have also been implicated in the maintenance of an allodynic state once it becomes established (Rao et al., 2008).

Multiple studies of patients with fibromyalgia have shown that the cerebrospinal fluid has three times the normal amount of substance P, a pain-facilitating substance. Additionally, nerve growth factor is elevated in patients with fibromyalgia, which results in altered sensory processing (Bennett, 2002). Other reductions in spinal cord fluid substances are serotonin, norepinephrine, and Dopamine, which suggests a connection to the depression associated with fibromyalgia.

The descending pain pathways may also be affected in patients with fibromyalgia. In some studies of patients with fibromyalgia, dysregulation of the descending pain pathways has been noted. This would allow painful stimuli to continue to be produced, with few if any blocking or braking mechanisms to control pain.

There are also differences in patients with fibromyalgia and control patients when functional magnetic resonance imaging was used. These images suggested that areas of painful peripheral stimuli produced increased blood flow to both groups of patients, but it occurred more quickly in patients with fibromyalgia. This means that the patients with fibromyalgia did not experience increased pain, but rather had a much faster onset of pain.

In one of the newest areas for fibromyalgia research, glial cells, a part of the support system for the nervous system, have been found to have new dimensions. The glial cells that surround pain neurons can enhance and alter the signaling and perception of pain. This is a relatively virgin area of research for fibromyalgia that may yield new information that will be helpful in determining how the pain of fibromyalgia is produced.

Assessment Tools

There are two common assessment tools that are used with patients with fibromyalgia. The Fibromyalgia Impact Questionnaire (FIQ) assesses health status in patients with fibromyalgia. The format is a short 10-item survey that asks questions about physical functioning, work status, depression, anxiety, sleep, pain, stiffness, and fatigue. To score the FIQ, each of the 10 questions has a maximum value of 10. The values of the 10 questions are combined to yield an overall score. The higher the score, the greater the impact of FMS on the patient.

Because the FIQ has a short and easy-to-use format, there is little patient burden with using it as a baseline and monitoring tool.

In a studies with tramadol using the FIQ, patients reported decreased pain scores and increased functionality, as measured with the FIQ (Burckhardt, Clark, & Bennett, 1991).

The Patient Global Impression of Change is used as a monitoring tool for patients to determine medication or intervention effectiveness. The tool consists of seven levels: very much improved; to 4, no change; to 7, very much worse. The positive scores are 1–3, and the negative scores are 5–7. The scoring of the tool is very subjective and based on the patient's impression of health status.

Treatment Options

There are a wide variety of medications being used to treat the pain and other elements of FMS. The three medications that have approval from the U.S. Food and Drug Administration for treating fibromyalgia pain are:

- pregabalin (Lyrica)—150–225 mg twice per day
- duloxetine (Cymbalta)—60 mg per day
- milnacipran (Savella)—50 mg twice a day (Mease et al., 2009)

The action of pregabalin, an anticonvulsant medication, is to bind to the alpha-2-delta subunit on a neuron with the resulting limitation of calcium influx, decreasing neuronal activity. It also affects the production of pain facilitators, substance P, and glutamate (Mease et al., 2009).

Duloxetine, an antidepressant medication, is a serotonin norepinephrine reuptake inhibitor. It works on the inhibitory pathway and modulates pain by allowing an increase in the available serotonin and norepinephrine (Mease et al., 2009).

Milnacipran, an antidepressant-type medication, has a selective serotonin reuptake inhibitor action. It also has a limited NMDA inhibition component (Mease et al., 2009.)

Each of the medications are started at lower doses and titrated up to the effective or maximum dose. The side effects of all of these medications are dose related. If the patient reports sedation, nausea, or dizziness, reducing the dose and titrating more slowly will facilitate tolerance of the medication. For mild sedation, the patients may need to take the medication at bedtime, rather than in the morning or during the day.

Other medications used to treat fibromyalgia that have evidence of efficacy are as follows:

- amitriptyline (Elavil) 25–50 mg/day—not recommended for older patients because of the potential for hypotension
- cyclobenzaprine (Flexeril) 10–30 mg/day at bedtime
- tramadol (Ultram) 200–300 mg/day
- fluoxetine (Prozac) 20–30 mg/day
- venlafaxine (Effexor) 37.5–300 mg/day (APS, 2005)

Other medications/drugs that show weak evidence for efficacy are as follows.

- S-adenosyl-methionine
- 5-hydroxytrptamine

Other medications/drugs that show no evidence for efficacy are as follows:

- Opioids
- Corticosteroids
- Nonsteroidal anti-inflammatory drugs
- Benzodiazepine-type medications
- Melatonin
- Calcitonin
- Thyroid hormone
- Guaifenesin
- Dehydroepiandrosterone (APS, 2005)

It is not uncommon to use a combination of medications to treat the various symptoms of FMS (Mease et al., 2009). The patient may be using pregabalin, duloxetine, or milnacipran for pain, along with a medication such as cyclobenzaprine as a muscle relaxant and to help promote sleep. When combining medications, use only one from a class, to avoid undesirable additive effects. For example, if you combine two drugs that boost serotonin levels, there is the potential for a serotonin syndrome to develop (Mease et al., 2009).

Nonpharmacologic Options

Treating fibromyalgia requires a combination of therapeutic options in addition to pharmacologic prescriptions. It is not a condition than lends itself to monotherapy. Using a combination of medications with integrative medicine techniques typically yields the best outcomes and provides the biggest benefit to the patient. The APS Fibromyalgia Guidelines (2005) recommend the addition of one or more of the following therapies:

- Cardiovascular exercise
- Cognitive behavioral therapies: relaxation, goal setting, problem solving, pace setting
- Patient education
- Multidisciplinary therapy

SUMMARY

When working with a patient with fibromyalgia, it is important to remember just how challenging the diagnostic process may have been for the patient. As a consequence, patient feelings about health care providers may be mixed. Working with the patient to create a trusting relationship and working collaboratively to establish a treatment regimen will help the patient understand the value of using a variety of integrative techniques, in addition to following the recommended medication regimen.

It is very encouraging that science has taken another look at the sources of fibromyalgia pain and has new information related to FMS being a neuropathic pain syndrome. Research on the function of glial cells and enhanced wind-up phenomenon will lead to a better understanding of what is causing the pain that patient's experience. As this information develops, there will be opportunities for treating the pain and ancillary symptoms of the syndrome with medications and techniques that will help restore the quality of life that these patients are seeking.

Jane Jones is a 35-year-old college student. She has returned to school to retrain for an occupation that does not require a lot of physical strength and endurance. She has chosen a teaching track in which she will teach art and art history to junior college students. She has been diagnosed with fibromyalgia and needs to have a less strenuous and stressful way to support herself. Her last job in retail left her feeling totally fatigued and worn out after a day of unpacking boxes and lifting clothing up onto racks. She was also required to stand for hours and run a cash register.

You ask Jane about her fibromyalgia and she tells you, "Well, it took 5 years for me to even get a diagnosis. I was going to my primary care doctor, who sent me to a rheumatologist, and between the two of them they still were very puzzled. Finally, they just decided I had fibro and that was it. What I hate most about the fibro is what it has done to my life. I can't do what I want to do; the aching and pain really limit me. I can't even get a good night's sleep. I am awake all night and just cat nap. I feel so tired all the time, and I fall asleep during the day. Some days I can't remember even the simplest things, and I really get frustrated because I know I am not that mentally off. Some of the treatments make me feel very irritable, and I usually just go home and hide out until I feel better. Some of the doctors thought this was all in my head, but I can tell you, I would certainly be willing to do anything to get my life back."

1. What combination of medication might work to help Jane sleep better and function at a higher level?
2. Are opioids appropriate for Jane?
3. What types of nonpharmacologic interventions would be good for Jane to try?
4. What is the most important thing that the health care provider must do to have a good outcome with Jane's treatment?
5. Is fibromyalgia a real illness?

REFERENCES

American Pain Society. (2005). *Guideline for the management of fibromyalgia syndrome in adults and children.* Glenview, IL: The American Pain Society.

Bennett, R. M. (2002). The rational management of fibromyalgia patients. *Rheumatic Diseases Clinics of North America, 28*(2), 1–16.

Burckhardt, C. S., Clark, S. R., & Bennett, R. M. (1991). The fibromyalgia impact questionnaire: Development and validation. *Journal of Rheumatology, 18*(5), 728–733.

D'Arcy, Y., & McCarberg, B. (2005). New fibromyalgia pain management recommendations. *The Nurse Practitioner Journal,* 31–40.

Hadhazy, V., Ezzo, J., Berman, B. M., Creamer, P., & Bausell, B. (2007). Mind and body therapy for fibromyalgia. *The Cochrane Collaboration, Cochrane Musculoskeletal Group,* 4.

Mease, P., Berney, S., Arnold, L., Clark, M., Goldenberg, D., Griffing, G., . . . Schur, P. (2009). *Fibromyalgia diagnostic and treatment challenges: Results from a recent summit of fibromyalgia experts.* Retrieved from http://cme.medscape.com

Rao, S., Gendreau, J., & Krentzler, J. (2008). Understanding the fibromyalgia syndrome. *Psychopharmacology Bulletin, 40*(4), 24–56.

Wolfe, F., Smythe, H. A., Yunus, M. B., Bennett, R. M., Bombardier, C., . . . Goldenberg, D. L. (1990). The American College of Rheumatology 1990 criteria for the classification of fibromyalgia report of the multicenter criteria committee. *Arthritis and Rheumatism, 33,* 160–172. Retrieved from http://www.rheumatology.org/practice/clinical/classification/fibromyalgia/1990_Criteria_for_Classification_Fibro.pdf

ADDITIONAL RESOURCES

Arnold, L. M., Rosen, A., Pritchett, Y. L., D'Souza, D. N., Goldenstein, D. J., . . . Iyengar, S. (2005). A randomized, double-blind, placebo-controlled trial of duloxetine in the treatment of women with fibromyalgia with or without a major depressive disorder. *Pain*, *119*(1–3), 5–15.

Arnold, L. M., Goldenberg, D. L., Stanford, S. B., Lalonde, J. K., Sandhu, H. S., . . . Keck, P. E. (2007). Gabapentin in the treatment of fibromyalgia: A randomized, double-blind, placebo-controlled multicenter trial. *Arthritis and Rheumatism*, *56*(4), 1336–1344.

Aryeh, A., Pillinger, M., Solitar, B., & Abeles, M. (2007). Narrative review: The pathophysiology of fibromyalgia. *Annals of Internal Medicine*, *146*, 726–734.

Crofford, L. J., Rowbotham, M. C., Mease, P. J., Russell, I. J., Dworkin, R. H., & Crobin, A. E. (2005). Pregabalin for the treatment of fibromyalgia syndrome: Results of a randomized, double-blind, placebo-controlled trial. *Arthritis and Rheumatism*, *52*(4), 1264–1273.

Gracely, R. H., Petzke, F., Wolf, J. M., & Clauw, D. J. (2002). Functional magnetic resonance imaging evidence of augmented pain processing in fibromyalgia. *Arthritis and Rheumatism*, *46*, 1333–1343.

Holdcraft, L. C., Assefi, N., & Buchwald, D. (2003). Complementary and alternative medicine in fibromyalgia and related syndromes. *Best Practice and Research in Clinical Rheumatology*, *17*(4), 667–683.

Karjalainen, K., Malmivaara, A., vanTulder, M., Roine, R., Jauhiainen, M., & Hurri, H. B. (2007). Multidisciplinary rehabilitation for fibromyalgia and musculoskeletal pain in working-age adults. *The Cochrane Collaboration, Cochrane Musculoskeletal Group*, 4.

Rooks, D., Gautam, S., Romeling, M., Cross, M., Stratigakis, D., Evans, B., . . . Katz, J. (2007). Group exercise, education, and combination self-management in women with fibromyalgia: A randomized trial. *Archives of Internal Medicine*, *167*(20), 2192–2200.

Rossy, L. A., Buckelew, S., Dorr, N., Hagglund, K., Thayer, J., McIntosh, M., . . . Johnson, J. (1999). A meta-analysis of fibromyalgia treatment interventions. *Annals of Behavioral Medicine*, *21*(2), 180–191.

Wallace, D. J., & Clauw, D. J. (2005). *Fibromyalgia and other central pain syndromes*. Philadelphia, PA: Lippincott Williams & Wilkins.

14

Headaches

OVERVIEW

There are four types of primary headaches classified by the International Headache Society. They are as follows:

- Migraine, with and without aura
- Chronic daily headache (CDH; e.g., tension-type headache [TTH])
- Cluster headache
- Other primary headaches (e.g., exertional headaches, hypertension-related headaches) (Silberstein et al., 2005)

Each of these headache types has diagnostic criteria and recommended treatments. Most patients who seek care for headache pain have a headache type that is chronic and has elements that are disruptive to their lifestyle and functionality. Many patients feel that the headache pain has a significant impact on the patient's personal life, relationships, and ability to work. The cyclical nature of some of the headache types contributes to patients fearing the unexpected recurrence of the headache at an inopportune time, when they really need to be able to function at full capacity. The disabling characteristic of the headache pain is something that patients learn to expect and fear.

When treating a patient who presents with a headache, all other sources of head pain should be considered and ruled out.

These conditions include brain tumor and other anatomic abnormalities such as Chari I malformations and syringomyelia, infection such as meningitis, and injuries such as subarachnoid bleed. Using magnetic resonance imaging (MRI), computed tomography, lumbar puncture, and electromyography testing can help to rule out other causes of headache and help with the diagnosis of migraine headache (American Society for Pain Management Nursing [ASPMN], 2009).

To diagnose a patient with headache, begin with a complete history and physical examination that delineates the clinical features and presentation of the headache. Seek information on how often the headaches occur, on triggers, and on pain type. Include a description of when the patient had the first headache, location severity, quality, frequency, duration, and what techniques relieve the pain. Ask about any family members who may have similar complaints. Take a complete medication history, including those medications that have been tried and found both effective and ineffective—include dose and length of time used here. Identify any accompanying symptoms, such as nausea or photophobia, or any triggering symptoms, such a specific food or smells. Ask the patient about the use of any types of nonpharmacologic interventions, such as self-hypnosis or relaxation techniques.

For the physical examination, conduct a full neurologic workup, including a funduscopic assessment, cranial nerves, reflexes, and muscle strength, noting neurologic impairment. Ask the patient about any changes in speech, memory, or mental status. As a final point, ask the patient about how the headache affects functionality, ability to work, sleep, or interpersonal interactions. Once the examination is complete and the diagnosis is made, the patients will need education of how best to prevent and treat the headache type he or she is experiencing.

Of the four major types of primary headache, perhaps the most discussed is the migraine headache. There is a great deal of literature on the topic. Migraineurs and CDH patients account for a high proportion of the total headache populations. Cluster headaches and other primary headaches, such as exertional headaches, account for far less of the headache population.

MIGRAINE HEADACHES

In the general population, the prevalence of migraine is 25% for women and 7.5% for men (Pringsheim, Davenport, & Dodick, 2008). In approximately 70% to 80% of migraineurs, there is a positive family history of migraine (Kolb-Lucas, 2008). The greatest incidence of migraines is between the ages of 25 and 55 years, affecting the highly productive middle-age time period.

Migraine headaches are broadly classed as:

- Migraine without aura
- Migraine with aura (Goadsby, 2006)

An *aura* associated with migraine is described as a symptom or set of symptoms that occur before a migraine attack. An aura occurs in approximately 20% of all migraines (Kolb-Lucas, 2008). The aura can be experienced as flashing lights, halos, double vision, or blind spots (scotoma) that the patient sees before the headache symptoms begin. Other more neurologically related symptoms include paresthesia, hemiplegia, aphasia, or vertigo (ASPMN, 2009; Kolb-Lucas, 2008). The aura symptoms commonly develop more than 5 to 20 minutes before the migraine and last approximately 20 minutes (ASPMN, 2009).

Common specific triggers for migraine headaches can include:

- Hormonal changes in women
- Foods such as pickled, preserved, or fermented products, aged cheese, salami, and freshly baked breads; alcohol, caffeinated beverages, caffeine withdrawal; fruits, nuts, and chocolate
- Stress
- Sensory stimuli
- Changes in sleep-wake patterns
- Changes in environment
- Medications

Physical triggers for migraine can be more diverse and more specialized to individual patients and include lack of sleep, too much sleep, illness, emotional stress, strong odors, weather, and seasonal changes (Kolb-Lucas, 2008).

A migraine headache typically includes five different stages:

- Prodrome—may occur well ahead of the headache—food cravings can occur
- Aura (if present)—as described above
- Headache phase—pain lasts for 24–72 hours
- Termination phase—head pain gradually resolving
- Postdrome phase—fatigue, irritability, muscle pain, or sleepiness that can last for a few days (Kolb-Lucas, 2008)

The headache itself is thought to be caused by vasodilatation and inflammatory responses. Activation of the nerve fibers innervating the dura mater are thought to produce the headache pain associated with increased intracranial pain of migraine (Pietrobon & Striessnig, 2003; Strassman, Raymond, & Burstein, 1996; Waeber & Moskowitz, 2005). Mast cells governing the immune response are associated with the inflammatory response and are located near blood vessels and afferent nociceptive neurons, implicating the cells in the creation of the pain from migraine headache (Levy et al., 2007). As the mast cells degranulate in response to the activation of the meningeal nociceptors, this is thought to prolong the headache and activate additional pain nociceptors in the spinal trigeminal nucleus (Levy et al., 2007).

The neurotransmitters involved in this process include calcitonin-gene-related peptide, neurokinin A, and substance P (Kolb-Lucas, 2008; Levy et al., 2007). Serotonin receptors produce an inflammatory response that further exacerbates the pain. The actual sensation of pain is produced by stimulation of the thalamus (Kolb-Lucas, 2008). Although the full mechanisms of migraine production are still not fully understood, the growing body of science in this area demonstrates that the process is complex and multifaceted.

Migraine Without Aura

The typical migraine without aura has specific characteristics that include five migraine attacks lasting at least 4–72 hours, with at least two of the following features:

- Unilateral location
- Moderate to severe pain intensity
- Pulsating
- Aggravated by routine activity

During the attack, two or more of the following symptoms are associated with migraine:

- Nausea
- Vomiting
- Photophobia
- Phonophobia
- Osmophobia (Silberstein et al., 2005)

Migraine With Aura

Migraine with aura has a particular set of symptoms that the patient regularly experiences before the onset of the headache. These include either visual or sensory symptoms. Migraine with aura has specific criteria, including the following:

- Headache that has the same elements as migraine without aura
- Presence of aura
- No permanent effects of the headache once the postdrome occurs

Menstrual migraine headaches are a women's pain syndrome that affects 50% to 60% of female migraine patients (Brandes, 2006). Menstrual migraine may occur with or without aura, but for purposes of classification, the International Headache Society describes menstrual migraine as a migraine headache without aura. In addition, the menstrual migraine occurs exclusively on day 1+/−2 of menstruation in at least 2 of 3 menstrual cycles (Silberstein et al., 2005). The cause of menstrual migraine is the variation in estrogen levels that normally occur with the menstrual cycle.

Treatment options for migraine headache include the use of nonpharmacologic treatments thought to reduce pain by 35% to 50%, such as:

- Biofeedback therapy
- Cognitive behavioral therapy
- Acupuncture
- Relaxation techniques
- Cooling pads
- Ginger

Medication options include:

- Abortive: triptan medication, nonsteroidal anti-inflammatory drugs, ergotamine, dihydroergotamine, butorphanol tartrate, Midrin, Fiorinal
- Prophylaxis: amitriptyline, propranolol, timolol, divalproex sodium, methylsergide
- Treatment: Moderate symptoms can be helped with triptan medications, such as sumatriptan, but use caution with patients who have uncontrolled hypertension or coronary artery disease. Opioids should be reserved for severe pain, coupled with medications such as metoclopramide for nausea and vomiting.

There are mixed reviews on the use of oral contraceptives and botulinum toxin injection. Oral contraceptives can worsen the migraine headaches in younger women (MyMigraineConnection.com, 2006). The recommendation for botulinum toxin injections is mixed. ASPMN (2009) makes the recommendation to use the injections, but the the U.S. Food and Drug Administration has issued a warning for botulinum toxin injections, because there is the potential for the injection to spread beyond the desired location.

CHRONIC DAILY HEADACHE: TENSION-TYPE HEADACHE

Patients with CDHs account for about 4% to 5% of the general patient population but constitute a large percentage (80%) of patients who are seen in specialty clinics for headache (Dodick & Saper, 2003).

Many patients with CDH (78%) also have chronic-transformed migraine (Dodick & Saper, 2003).

Diagnostic criteria for CDH include:

- Headache occurs at least 15 days per month.
- Headaches last for longer than 4 hours per day (Dodick & Saper, 2003).

What causes a CDH? The average CDH patient has a history of long-term episodic migraine, with headaches that gradually increase in frequency. There can be a family history of depression, anxiety, or alcoholism (Dodick & Saper, 2003).

Although the true cause of CDH is still being investigated, there are some common theories that are considered to be valid for determining the source of CDH pain. Pathophysiologic mechanisms that are considered to contribute to CDH include:

- Medication overuse
- Genetic alterations in the central brain and pain-modulating systems
- Deficiencies or excesses in neurotransmitter systems
- Stress or trauma
- Brain stem changes related to free-radical damage and iron deposition (Dodick & Saper, 2003)

No matter what the cause of the CDH, the effect can be very disruptive to the patient. For patients who are overusing medications, trying to taper and stop the overuse medication can result in a withdrawal headache that will also cause pain. The vicious circle of medication use for headache and trying to manage the medication withdrawal can be quite challenging. Prophylactic treatment should start prior to the withdrawal of any medications. Medications that can be used during this period as preventative treatment include tricyclic antidepressants, beta blockers, antiepileptic drugs, and ergot derivatives. Suggested measures to manage the withdrawal headache include:

- Clonidine for opioid withdrawal
- Temporary substitution of phenobarbital for butalbital to avoid seizures or other serious withdrawal symptoms
- Intravenous dihydroergotamine for headache relief (Ward, 2004)

Tapering and replacement of medications can take as long as 1 to 3 months. Careful monitoring of headache symptoms and adverse effects is needed to ensure maximum pain control and symptom management.

Treatment options for CDH are varied, and the overuse aspect of the condition limits some of the available options. The use of medication to treat the pain of CDH should be to target pain relief and provide additional support for treating flare migraine headaches when they occur.

The goals of treatment for CDH include the following:

1. Design a treatment plan that combines a variety of approaches that

   - Minimize symptomatology
   - Reduce disability
   - Improve quality of life

2. Provide follow-up care for long-term headache management

   - Reassess and revise treatment plan and assess for goal achievement
   - Reevaluate patient needs and track headache patterns

3. Recognize the need for referral to specialists (Ward, 2004)

Tension-Type Headache

TTH is a form of CDH. It is a category that headaches fall into when all other types of headaches have been ruled out. The TTH is diagnosed when the headache occurs 15 days per month for at least 3 months (ASPMN, 2009).

For a headache to be classed as a TTH, it should meet the following criteria:

- Nonpulsating tightening or pressing sensation
- Mild or moderate intensity
- Bilateral location
- Not induced by physical activity (ASPMN, 2009)

The treatment options for TTH are similar to those for CDH.

CLUSTER HEADACHE

The cluster headache is just as it is titled: headaches that occur in groups over a period of time. These headaches can occur daily for weeks or months and then a remission or attack-free period occurs. Cluster headaches are more prevalent in women than men, and the overall occurrence rate is 0.1% to 0.4% in the general population. Onset is fairly young, with the mean age being late 20s. Cluster periods can last for 2 months and range in length from 4–15 weeks. Interestingly, cluster headaches tend to occur at the same time of day and the same time of year.

Criteria for cluster headaches include:

- Unilateral location
- Extremely severe pain around the orbital and temporal regions
- Headache lasting for 15 minutes to 3 hours
- Pain accompanied by autonomic symptoms, such as lacrimation, nasal congestion, miosis, ptosis, and facial flushing (ASPMN, 2009)

The cause of cluster headaches is associated with activation of the trigeminal vascular and cranial parasympathetic pathways, with an increase in calcitonin gene-related peptide and vasoactive intestinal peptide (Goadsby, 2006). Nitroglycerin can precipitate a cluster headache, leading to the belief that increase levels of nitric oxide are also implicated in the production of a cluster headache (Dodick & Saper, 2003).

Treatment options for cluster headaches include the following:

- Application of oxygen of 6–7 liters for 15 minutes
- Triptans
- Intranasal lidocaine
- ergotamine derivatives
- gabapentin

Preventative options for treating cluster headache include the following:

- lithium
- verapamil
- ergotamine

- dihydroergotamine
- Corticosteroids

There are a variety of surgical interventions that can also be used to treat cluster headaches. Most involve blockade, rhizotomy of the trigeminal nerve, and neuromodulation (ASPMN, 2009).

OTHER PRIMARY HEADACHES

There are a variety of primary headaches that are associated with a specific trigger mechanism. These headaches include:

- Exertional headache
- Hypertension-related headache
- Thunderclap headache, which has acute onset and mimics ruptured cerebral aneurysm
- Primary cough headache
- Primary headache associated with sexual activity
- Primary stabbing headache
- Hemicrania continua, a persistent unilateral headache (ASPMN, 2009; Silberstein et al., 2005)

Each of these headaches has an associated cause and treatment options that are similar to those of other headache types.

No matter what the cause of the headache the patient experiences, headache pain has a significant impact on the patient's personal life and functional ability. For headaches with prophylaxis and abortive treatment option, the patient should be provided with medications that are effective to reduce the occurrence and frequency of the headache. Side effects of the headache, such as nausea and vomiting, should be treated with effective antiemetics.

The treatment for headaches in general does not rely solely on medications. There are many nonpharmacologic options, such as relaxation and biofeedback, that can help headache patients control their headaches. By combining medications and nonpharmacologic options, patients with headache can help to control the occurrence, severity, and frequency of headaches. This in turn will help the patient to achieve a better quality of life and a more normal lifestyle.

Carol Ann is a 35-year-old patient who reports repeated headaches. They seem to come at regular intervals, and she reports the pain intensity as severe. She is currently taking Oxycontin, 40 mg three times a day with oxycodone for breakthrough pain. She is also taking an antiemetic for her nausea. When you speak to Carol Ann about her headaches she tells you, "I have tried all those other medications. Nothing seems to work for me and now the pain medication doesn't seem to be controlling the pain either. Ibuprofen doesn't work, and all those other pain medications are too weak for the pain. My mother had these headaches, too. She used to get them around her period, and then we all had to be quiet and help out until she got better. Mine come around my period, too. I hate to see my kids going through I did as kid when my Mom had her headaches. Is there anything you can do to help me?"

Questions to Consider

1. What type of headache does Carol Ann have?
2. Are opioids the best treatment for her headache?
3. What treatment options would be better for treating the pain of Carol Ann's headache?
4. Is there anything you could prescribe that would decrease the frequency of the headaches or stop them from occurring?
5. Are there options for using nonpharmacologic treatments?

REFERENCES

American Society for Pain Management Nursing. (2009). *Core curriculum for pain management nursing* (2nd ed.). Lanexa, KS: American Society for Pain Management Nursing.

Brandes, J. L. (2006). The influence of estrogen on migraine. *Journal of the American Medical Society, 295*(15), 1824–1830.

Dodick, D. W., & Saper, J. (2003). Cluster and chronic daily headache. *Neurology, 60*(Suppl. 2), S31–S37.

Goadsby, P. J. (2006). Primary neurovascular headache. In S. B. McMahon & M. Koltzenberg (Eds.). *Textbook of pain* (5th ed., pp. 851–874). Philadelphia, PA: Elsevier.

Kolb-Lucas, K. (2008). Strategies for treating migraines. *Nursing 2008, 33*(5), 32cc4–32cc6.

Levy, D., Burstein, R., Kainz, V., Jakubowski, M., & Strassman, A. M. (2007). Mast cell degranulation activates a pain pathway underlying migraine headache. *Pain, 130,* 166–176.

Pietrobon, D., & Striessnig, J. (2003). Neurobiology of migraine. *Nature Reviews Neuroscience, 4,* 386–398.

Pringsheim, T., Davenport, W. J., & Dodick, D. (2008). Acute treatment and prevention of menstrually related migraine headache: Evidence-based review. *Neurology, 70,* 1555–1563.

Silberstein S. D., Olesen, J., Bousser, M., Diener, H., Dodick, D., First, M., … Steiner, T. J. (2005). International classification of headache disorders, 2nd edition (ICHD-II)—revision of criteria for 8.2 Medication—overuse headache. *Cephalalgia, 25*(6), 460–465.

Strassman, A. M., Raymond, S. A., & Burstein, R. (1996). Sensitization of meningeal sensory neurons and the origin of headaches. *Nature, 384*, 560–564.

Waeber, C., & Moskowitz, M. A. (2005). Migraine as an inflammatory disorder. *Neurology, 64*, S9–S15.

Ward, M. (2004). Treatment of primary headache: Chronic daily headache. In *Standards of care for headache diagnosis and treatment* (pp. 73–80). Chicago, IL: National Headache Foundation. Retrieved from www.guideline.gov

ADDITIONAL RESOURCES

D'Arcy, Y. (2009). Finding relief for menstrually related migraines. *The Nurse Practitioner, 34*(7), 7–9.

Hu, X. H., Markson, L. E., Lipton, R. B., Stewart, W. F., & Berger, M. L. (1999). Burden of migraine in the United States: Disability and economic costs. *Archives of Internal Medicine, 59*, 813–818.

Martin, V. T. (2004). Menstrual migraine: A review of prophylactic therapies. *Current Pain and Headache Reports, 8*, 229–237.

Pietrobon, D. (2005). Migraine: New molecular mechanisms. *Neuroscientist, 11*, 373–386.

Stovner, L. J., Hagen, K. Jensen, R., Katsarava Z., Lipton, R., et al. (2007). The global burden of headache: A documentation of headache prevalence and disability worldwide. *Cephalalgia, 27*, 193–210.

Tepper, S. (2006). Tailoring management strategies for the patient with menstrual migraine: Focus on prevention and treatment. *Headache, 46*(Suppl. 2), S61–S68.

V

Managing Neuropathic Pain Syndromes

15

Overview of Neuropathic Pain

NEUROPATHIC PAIN

Neuropathic pain is one of the most difficult chronic pain conditions to treat. Patients can suffer for many years without knowing what the pain they are experiencing is caused by or what treatment options are available. Patients will describe the pain as painful aching that may worsen at night in their legs, as a painful numbness in their hands, or as any number of strange sensations that are painful. What they will also say is that most of the typical treatments for pain, such as medications or topical creams or balms, or comfort measures such as ice or heat really do not seem to help the pain. This leaves the patient with a feeling of hopelessness related to getting any help for treating this type of pain that has a significant impact on his or her quality of life.

In general, neuropathic pain is caused by damage to nerves in either the peripheral nervous system or the central nervous system. The damage can be from a number of causes: infections, trauma, and chronic illness. The International Association for the Study of Pain defines neuropathic pain as "pain initiated or caused by a primary lesion or dysfunction in the nervous system that disrupts impulse transmission and modulation of sensory input" (Polomano & Farrar, 2006). Clifford Wolfe has described neuropathic pain as "pain that has no breaking mechanisms." It can be a self-perpetuating entity related to ongoing inflammatory effect that continues to sustain the pain.

The fact that the pain not only is caused by a dysfunction of the nervous system but also affects the ability of the body to detect sensory input or augment sensory input is very important. This can help to explain some of the patient presentations and patient complaints with the condition that seem difficult to interpret.

> *Clinical Pearl*
>
> Neuropathic pain may be more difficult to diagnose because it can present as a single condition or it can be combined with other pain presentations, such as acute, chronic, or other neuropathic pain conditions. For example, patients with a diabetic neuropathy may also have osteoarthritis or be seen in the surgical setting.

Neuropathic pain differs from nociceptive pain in that it is caused by damage to nerves, not to muscles or tendons. For neuropathic pain, nociceptive input from peripheral receptors is not always required. In the centrally mediated neuropathic pain syndromes, such as poststroke pain or complex regional pain syndrome (CRPS), sensory input is not required for the pain to be produced and persist. Neuropathic pain is also of higher intensity than the injury would indicate.

Common causes of neuropathic pain include the following:

- Nerve damage during surgical procedures (e.g., postmastectomy pain syndrome, postthoracotomy pain syndrome, phantom limb pain, and nerve entrapment conditions, such as posthernioraphy pain or posthysterectomy nerve entrapment syndrome)
- Chronic illness or conditions (e.g., painful diabetic neuropathy [PDN])
- Treatment-related neuropathies (e.g., chemotherapy-related neuropathies)
- Infective neuropathies (e.g., acquired immunodeficiency syndrome/human immunodeficiency virus [HIV], postherpetic neuralgia [PHN])
- Toxic neuropathies (e.g., ethyl alcohol, heavy metal)

As with many chronic pain conditions, no matter what the cause of the neuropathy, the treatment is aimed at controlling the symptoms. The chronicity of neuropathic pain can be defeating for both the patients and the practitioner trying to treat their pain. In a qualitative study in which focus groups of patients with neuropathic pain discussed their feelings about the condition, the patients felt that the usual medications used to treat the pain were not very effective and had unpleasant side effects (Closs et al., 2007). Complementary methods had little effect, and the patients found that resting or retreating was most helpful. The patients all expressed frustration with trying to find a way to control the pain. They reported experiencing many failed attempts, followed by continued searching for help with the pain (Closs et al., 2007). This repeated searching for answers and help can lead to the patient being labeled as someone who is "doctor shopping."

Some patients who do get a diagnosis feel more reassured when they know the name of the pain they are experiencing (Staats et al., 2004). It helps a patient to know what the condition they have is called. It does not matter that the outcome has not changed, but knowing what to call the pain complaint will give some measure of comfort to the patient. The uncertainty about the pain is more destructive than knowing what the condition is.

THE PATHOPHYSIOLOGY OF NEUROPATHIC PAIN

Patients who have neuropathic pain will report consistent pain that can be painfully numb. The pain may also have a paroxysmal component. Extreme sensitivity to cold air passage over the affected area and burning sensations are also common. The descriptors that patients use for the pain are the best means of diagnosing the pain complaint as neuropathic. These descriptors include:

- Painful numbness
- Tingling
- Burning
- Shooting

- Pins and needles
- Strange painful sensations (Irving, 2005)

Typically, the pain the patient experiences from a neuropathic condition is worse at night, especially with conditions such as PDN. It is important for the health care provider to question the patient who is suspected of having a neuropathic source for their pain about the type of pain they are having; if anything causes the pain, such as movement, pressure, or differences in temperature; and if there are times of day when the pain is worse.

Physiologically, neuropathic pain has been described as pain without a braking mechanism. The pain stimulus is sustained by a collection of pain-facilitating substances, such as bradykinin, that are recruited to create the pain and continue and expand the effects of the pain stimulus. Once the nerve injury occurs, what is called an "inflammatory soup" of pain facilitators, such as substance P, hydrogen ions, interleukin-1(beta), nerve growth factor, prostaglandins, histamine, bradykinin, adenosine-5'-triphosphate, and tumor necrosis factor, are activated to help sustain an inflammatory cycle that continues and spreads the effects of the condition (Irving, 2005).

Once the physiologic changes start, the effects on the sodium channels that are related to pain transmission take place. For a normal transmission of pain, primary sodium channels on neurons are activated. The accumulation of the pain facilitators in neuropathic pain activate secondary sodium channels on neurons that produce a slower activation and are related to pain production. When nerve damage occurs, both types of sodium channels are activated, causing a hyperexcitable neuronal state with the potential for ectopic neuronal discharge (Irving, 2005).

Two of the most common conditions associated with the hyperexcitability of the neuronal system are allodynia and hyperalgesia:

- Allodynia is perception of pain caused by a normally nonpainful stimulus, such as light touch or hugs.
- Hyperalgesia is an increased sensation of pain in response to a normally painful stimulus, such as intravenous needle insertion (Staats et al., 2004).

Other terms that are used to describe neuropathic pain are paresthesia, dysesthesia, and numbness:

- Paresthesias are abnormal spontaneous sensations, such as burning tingling, pins, and needles.
- Numbness is a descriptor applied by patients to a feeling of heaviness, weakness, or deadness in the affected area of the body. It is also described as painful numbness.
- Dysesthesia is a response where an unpleasant sensation is produced by normal sensation.

Diagnosing neuropathic pain is a challenge for health care practitioners. Although the pain descriptors the patient uses are helpful is discriminating neuropathic pain from other types of pain, the patient also presents with confounding symptoms as well. Patients with neuropathic pain can also present with not only pain but also insomnia, anorexia, anxiety, depression, physical inactivity, and a diminished quality of life (Irving, 2005). Because neuropathic pain is a more complex presentation than a nociceptive type of pain, such as an ankle sprain, the treatment is also more complex and may take weeks or months to be effective. Making a diagnosis of neuropathic pain and selecting a treatment means that the patient with neuropathic pain will need closer follow-up and careful titration of medication with careful assessment of adverse effects, such as sedation, nausea, or constipation. However, a careful examination of the patient's pain that reveals a neuropathic component can help to ease the burden of care for both the patient and health care professional if it is identified early on in the evaluation process, and the correct medication regimen selected.

PREVALENCE OF NEUROPATHIC PAIN

Neuropathic pain is much more common than previously suspected. The overall prevalence of neuropathic pain is thought to be approximately 1,765,000 people, excluding those patients with lower back pain radiculopathy (Irving, 2005). If the back pain patients were included, the numbers would be significantly higher at 3,865,000 patients.

The types of neuropathic pain syndromes are generally organized into peripheral neuropathic pain syndromes and central neuropathic pain syndromes. The peripheral neuropathic pain syndromes are further classified into categories, including the following:

- Painful diabetic neuropathy (600,000 patients)
- Postherpetic neuralgia (500,000 patients)
- Cancer associated (200,000 patients)
- HIV associated (100,000 patients)
- Phantom limb pain (50,000 patients)

The central neuropathic pain syndromes are further classified into the following categories:

- Spinal cord injury (120,000 patients)
- CRPS I and II (100,000 patients)
- Poststroke (30,000 patients) (Irving, 2005)

Although these numbers seem large, they will continue to grow. War-related injuries to members of the armed services requiring amputations will increase the number of patients with phantom limb pain. The increase in obesity and resultant diabetes will increase the number of patients who have the potential to develop PDN. Additionally, previously unrecognized cases of neuropathic pain will increase the overall number of cases as health care providers become more proficient at assessing and identifying pain as having a neuropathic cause rather than nociceptive pain.

The impact of these syndromes on the lives of the patients who have them is multifaceted. One article that reviewed the impact of neuropathic pain on health-related quality of life reported that the presence and severity of neuropathic pain is associated with the potential for diminished quality of life in several important domains. These included the following:

- Physical functioning
- Emotional functioning
- Sleep quality

- Role functioning
- Work and educational activities
- Social functioning

The higher the severity of pain, the more impact it had on these quality-of-life domains (Jensen, Chodroff, & Dworkin, 2007). This study also suggests that health care providers need to take a more in-depth and focused assessment of neuropathic pain that follows a biopsychosocial model rather than the more commonly used biomedical approach (Jensen et al., 2007). Given the deep-reaching effects of chronic neuropathic pain, it is incumbent on health care practitioners to become familiar with the type of syndromes and causes of neuropathic pain that are most common in today's health care practices.

ASSESSING NEUROPATHIC PAIN

There are some pain assessment tools that are specific for neuropathic pain. They are designed to evaluate the specific elements of a neuropathic pain condition. In clinical practice, a tool for diagnosing neuropathic pain may not be needed, but there are several that are specifically designed for assessing the patient with suspected neuropathic pain. The Neuropathic Pain Scale (NPS), the Leeds Neuropathic Pain Scale (S-LANSS), and the revised Short-Form McGill Pain Questionnaire-2 (SF-MPQ-2) are three tools that have been developed specifically to assess the neuropathic components of a pain complaint. The new revised SF-MPQ-2 has the ability to differentiate between a neuropathic pain and a non-neuropathic pain.

When assessing a neuropathic pain complaint, it is important to use not only a recognized pain scale but also a variety of physical tests. Subjecting the painful area to heat and cold and testing sensation with cotton wisps, manual pressure, pinprick, or alcohol wipes can help define the specific area of the pain and associated painful sensations. Once the affected area is determined, the health care provider can track the area to see if it becomes less sensitive or decreases in size.

Neuropathic Pain Scale

The NPS (Exhibit 15.1) was developed as a result of two research protocols in which pain descriptors were assessed for four different pain conditions: PHN, CRPS, PDN, and traumatic peripheral nerve injury. A second, more diverse group of patients being treated with either lidocaine or phentolamine infusions used the scale to rate their pain. Interestingly, the second protocol outcome identified a positive response for pain that was described as "unpleasant or deep." This finding led researchers to believe that the descriptors that are used by patients are really clues to the specific mechanisms that are producing the pain. More research is needed to correlate the various descriptors with individual mechanisms.

The NPS is a 10-item scale using an 11-point Likert-like rating scale where 0 indicates not sensitive, itchy, and dull, and 10 indicates the most sensitive, itchy, and dull.

It is a reliable and valid tool for measuring neuropathic pain, and it can also differentiate between nociceptive and neuropathic pain. The higher the score, the more intense the neuropathic pain.

In a study of chronic pain patients having a nociceptive or neuropathic pain condition, the NPS was used to differentiate the two pain types by score. The score of 5.53 was determined to be the cutoff point that delineated nociceptive from neuropathic type pain. Nociceptive pain types, such as myofascial syndrome, had a score of 3.81, whereas CRPS I and II had scores of 6.87 and 9.34, respectively. These results reinforce the original findings of higher NPS scores, indicating a neuropathic pain syndrome.

Advantages of the NPS are as follows:

- Two items that measure the global dimensions of pain intensity and pain unpleasantness
- One item that addresses the fluctuation of pain from constant with intermittent increases, that are intermittently constant with fluctuation
- Higher scores indicative of a pain that is more neuropathic
- Can measure the effects of treatments

Exhibit 15.1

NEUROPATHIC PAIN SCALE© (NPS©)

<u>Instructions</u>: There are several different aspects of pain which we are interested in measuring: pain **sharpness, heat/cold, dullness, intensity** overall **unpleasantness**, and **surface vs. deep** pain.

The distinction between these aspects of pain might be clearer if you think of taste. For example, people might agree on how <u>sweet</u> a piece of pie might be (the **intensity** of the sweetness) but some might enjoy it more if it were sweeter while others might prefer it to be less sweet. Similarly, people can judge the loudness of music and agree on what is more quiet and what is louder, but disagree on how it makes them feel. Some prefer quiet music and some prefer it more loud. In short, the <u>intensity</u> of a sensation is not the same as how it makes you feel. A sound might be unpleasant and still be quiet (think of someone grating their fingernails along a chalkboard). A sound can be quiet and "dull" or loud and "dull".

Pain is the same. Many people are able to tell the difference between many aspects of their pain: for example, <u>how much</u> it hurts, and <u>how unpleasant</u> or annoying it is. Although often the intensity of pain has strong influence on how unpleasant the experience of pain is, some people are able to experience more pain than others before they feel very bad about it.

There are scales for measuring different aspects of pain. For one patient, a pain might feel extremely hot, but not at all dull, while another patient may not experience any heat, but feel like their pain is very dull. We expect you to rate very high on some of the scales below, and very low on others. We want you to use the measures that follow to tell us exactly what you experience.

Place an "X" through the number that best describes your pain.

1. Please use the scale below to tell us how **intense** your pain is.

| No pain | 0 | 1 | 2 | 3 | 4 | 5 | 6 | 7 | 8 | 9 | 10 | The most **intense** pain sensation imaginable |

2. Please use the scale below to tell us how **sharp** your pain feels. Words used to describe "sharp" feelings include "like a knife", "like a spike", "like a spike", or "like jolts".

| Not sharp | 0 | 1 | 2 | 3 | 4 | 5 | 6 | 7 | 8 | 9 | 10 | The most **sharp** sensation imaginable ("like a knife") |

3. Please use the scale below to tell us how **hot** your pain feels. Words used to describe very hot pain include "burning" and "on fire".

| Not hot | 0 | 1 | 2 | 3 | 4 | 5 | 6 | 7 | 8 | 9 | 10 | The most **hot** sensation imaginable ("on fire") |

4. Please use the scale below to tell us how **dull** your pain feels. Words used to describe very dull pain include "like a dull toothache", "dull pain", and "like a bruise".

| Not dull | 0 | 1 | 2 | 3 | 4 | 5 | 6 | 7 | 8 | 9 | 10 | The most **dull** sensation imaginable |

5. Please use the scale below to tell us how **cold** your pain feels. Words used to describe very cold pain include "like ice" and "freezing".

| Not cold | 0 | 1 | 2 | 3 | 4 | 5 | 6 | 7 | 8 | 9 | 10 | The most **cold** sensation imaginable ("freezing") |

©GALER & JENSEN, 1997. All rights reserved. Please contact the MAPI Institute (http://www.mapiinstitute.com) to obtain permission to use the Neuropathic Pain Scale.

10-items NPS – US English

Note: From "Development and preliminary validation of a pain measure specific to neuropathic pain: The Neuropathic Pain Scale," by B. S. Galer and M. P. Jensen, 1997, *Neurology, 48*, pp. 332–338. Copyright 1997 by Lippincott Williams & Wilkins. Reprinted with permission.

(Continued)

(Continued)

6. Please use the scale below to tell us how **sensitive** your skin is to light touch or clothing. Words used to describe sensitive skin include "like sunburned skin", and "raw skin".

Not sensitive | 0 | 1 | 2 | 3 | 4 | 5 | 6 | 7 | 8 | 9 | 10 | The most **sensitive** sensation imaginable ("raw skin")

7. Please use the scale below to tell us how **itchy** your pain feels. Words used to describe itchy pain include "like poison oak" and "like a mosquito bite".

Not itchy | 0 | 1 | 2 | 3 | 4 | 5 | 6 | 7 | 8 | 9 | 10 | The most **itchy** sensation imaginable ("like poison oak")

8. Which of the following best describes the **time** quality of your pain? Please check only one answer.

( ) I feel a background pain <u>all of the time</u> **and** occasional flare-ups (break-through pain) <u>some of the time</u>.

Describe the background pain: _____

Describe the flare-up (break-through) pain: _____

( ) I feel a single type of pain <u>all the time</u>. Describe this pain: _____

( ) I feel a single type of pain only <u>sometimes</u>. Other times, I am pain free.

Describe this occasional pain: _____

9. Now that you have told us the different physical aspects of your pain, the different types of sensations, we want you to tell us overall how **unpleasant** your pain is to you. Words used to describe very unpleasant pain include "miserable" and "intolerable". Remember, pain can have a low intensity, but still feel extremely unpleasant, and some kinds of pain can have a high intensity but be very tolerable. With this scale, please tell us how **unpleasant** your pain feels.

Not unpleasant | 0 | 1 | 2 | 3 | 4 | 5 | 6 | 7 | 8 | 9 | 10 | The most **unpleasant** sensation imaginable ("intolerable")

10. Lastly we want you to give us an estimate of the severity of your <u>deep</u> versus <u>surface</u> pain. We want you to rate each location of pain separately. We realize that it can be difficult to make these estimates, and most likely it will be a "best guess", but please give us your best estimate.

HOW INTENSE IS YOUR *DEEP* PAIN?

No **deep** pain | 0 | 1 | 2 | 3 | 4 | 5 | 6 | 7 | 8 | 9 | 10 | The most **intense deep** pain sensation imaginable

HOW INTENSE IS YOUR *SURFACE* PAIN?

No **surface** pain | 0 | 1 | 2 | 3 | 4 | 5 | 6 | 7 | 8 | 9 | 10 | The most **intense surface** pain sensation imaginable

©GALER & JENSEN, 1997. All rights reserved. Please contact the MAPI Institute (http://www.mapiinstitute.com) to obtain permission to use the Neuropathic Pain Scale.

10-items NPS – US English

Note: From "Development and preliminary validation of a pain measure specific to neuropathic pain: The Neuropathic Pain Scale," by B. S. Galer and M. P. Jensen, 1997, *Neurology, 48*, pp. 332–338. Copyright 1997 by Lippincott Williams & Wilkins. Reprinted with permission.

Used with permission of the authors.

Disadvantages of the NPS are as follows:

- Data collected from chronic pain clinic patients that do not reflect the total experience of the larger patient population with neuropathic pain
- Validation study not randomized; double-blind construct
- Not all types of neuropathic pain complaints covered in the 11 items of the scale

S-LANSS is a self-administered survey format assessment tool to determine if pain is neuropathic. The main value to the S-LANSS is that it can be used to determine if a patient with chronic pain has a neuropathic element to the pain complaint. It measures similar indicators to the NPS, such as cold sensitivity, pain with pressure, and so forth. The higher the score, the more it indicates a neuropathic type of pain.

Advantages of the S-LANSS are as follows:

- Easy to use
- Self-administered survey format

Disadvantages of the S-LANSS are as follows:

- Less specificity and sensitivity when used in population studies
- Best suited as a screening tool rather than an assessment tool
- Used to screen pain for neuropathic component in chronic pain patients of all types

Short-Form McGill Pain Questionnaire-2 (SF-MPQ-2)

In the original McGill Pain Questionnaire used to assess pain in chronic pain patients, there is a list of 15 verbal descriptors rated on a 4-point scale, a visual analog scale for pain intensity, and verbal rating scales. The original scale established reliability and validity for measuring pain in chronic pain conditions. Although some chronic pain conditions are neuropathic, a tool that can distinguish both the pain of a chronic nociceptive condition and neuropathic pain is considered desirable.

The SF-MPQ was expanded by adding in nine symptoms that were indicative of neuropathic pain, and the 4-point rating scale was replaced with a 0- to 10-point rating scale. The new symptom descriptors that were added included squeezing pressure, piercing, itching, tingling pins and needles, numbness, pain caused by light touch, cold freezing, electric shock pain, and dullness. It was hoped that the changes would make it easier to determine the type of pain that the patient was experiencing.

The researchers used a variety of testing methods that included patient focus groups, a web-based survey for patients with chronic pain, and a clinical trial for patients with PDN. A total of 882 patients completed the SF-MPQ-2 pain assessment tool via the web survey, and 226 patients used the new tool in the PDN trial. In general, the SF-MPQ-2 was found to be both reliable and valid for measuring chronic pain and chronic neuropathic pain (Dworkin et al., 2009). It also has good support for four subscales in the tool that interpret continuous pain, intermittent pain, predominantly neuropathic pain, and affective descriptors (Dworkin et al.).

Advantages of the SF-MPQ-2 are as follows:

■ Can be used for all types of chronic pain, short format, and easy to use
■ Use of three different methods to determine reliability and validity
■ Has reliability and validity
■ Has four subscales that interpret continuous pain, intermittent pain, pain of neuropathic origin, and affective descriptors

Disadvantages of the SF-MPQ-2 are as follows:

■ It uses a web-survey format where patients have to self-declare as patients with chronic pain, with no confirmation.
■ The patients in the focus groups were selected patients who were receiving treatment at pain centers and as a group may not represent typical patients with chronic pain.

TREATMENT OPTIONS FOR NEUROPATHIC PAIN

There are a variety of treatment options for neuropathic pain. The most recent recommendations are included in the stepwise management of neuropathic pain from a guideline designed to direct medication and therapeutic choices using evidence-based recommendations (Exhibit 15.2). The guideline is available at www.guideline.gov.

Exhibit 15.2

Stepwise Pharmacologic Management of Neuropathic Pain (NP)

Step 1

- Assess pain and establish the diagnosis. Treat the cause if possible (or refer).
- Identify relevant comorbidities that might influence drug selection, dosage adjustment, or additional monitoring of therapy.
- Explain the diagnosis and treatment plan to the patient, and establish realistic expectations.

Step 2

- Initiate symptom treatment with one or more of the following:
  - A secondary amine tricyclic antidepressant or a selective serotonin and norepinephrine reuptake inhibitor
  - A selective (calcium channel alpha 2-sigma ligand) anticonvulsant, such as gabapentin or pregabalin
  - A topical lidocaine if the neuropathy and allodynia localized
  - Nonpharmacologic treatments as appropriate and acceptable to patient

Step 3

- Reassess pain, adverse effects and functioning frequently. Continue treatment with satisfactory response (often considered when pain reduced to <3/10).
- If partial pain relief (e.g., pain remains >4/10) and tolerable side effects, add another first-line medications.
- If no pain relief (e.g., <30% reduction) or intolerable side effects, switch to an alternative first-line medication.

Step 4

If trials of first-line medications alone and in combination fail, consider second- and third-line medications or referral to a pain specialist or multidisciplinary pain center.

Source: Adapted from Dworkin et al., 2009.

First-Line Medications

Tricyclic antidepressants (TCAs) have strong research support for use, Forty percent to 60% of patients report pain relief. They are especially useful for patients with PDN and PHN and those who have an element of depression in their overall presentation. These drugs are not benign and careful monitoring is needed. A baseline electrocardiography is recommended for patients older than 40 years to evaluate for the presence of conduction abnormalities. Adverse side effects include cardiotoxicity, confusion, urinary retention, orthostatic hypotension, weight gain, dry mouth, and constipation. Patients who have a history of cardiac ischemia, heart failure, conduction disorders, or arrhythmias should not use TCAs. They are also not recommended for older patients related to the potential for orthostatic hypotension.

Recommended antidepressant medications include the following:

■ *Amitriptyline hydrochloride (Elavil)*

Dosage: 10 to 25 mg at bedtime with a maximum dose of 50–150 mg daily. Increase dose cautiously and monitor for the side effects. Instruct patient to take the medication in the early evening to reduce the effect of early morning sedation.

Precaution: In the elderly amitriptyline not recommended due to incidence of early morning hypotension.

■ *Nortriptyline hydrochloride (Pamelor, Aventyl)*

Dosage: 25 mg by mouth at bedtime. Increase dose by 25 mg every 3–7 days to a maximum of 150 mg daily

Precaution: adjust dosages in elderly and adolescent patients

■ *Desipramine hydrochloride (Norpramin)*

Dosage: 25 mg by mouth at bedtime. Increase dose by 25 mg every 3–7 days to a maximum of 150 mg daily

Precautions: cardiac disease, glaucoma, suicide risk, seizure disorder, concomitant use of monoamine oxidase inhibitors

Selective serotonin norepinephrine reuptake inhibitors include the following:

■ **Duloxetine hydrochloride (Cymbalta)**

Dosage: 30 mg by mouth once daily. Increase to 60 mg once daily after 1 week; maximum dose 60 mg twice per day

Indication: useful for patients with PDN and has long-term data that support its use for PDN

Precautions: hepatic dysfunction, renal insufficiency, alcohol abuse, concomitant use of tramadol

■ **Venlafaxine hydrochloride (Effexor)**

Dosage: 37.5 mg by mouth once or twice daily. Increase by 75 mg each week to a maximum of 225 mg daily

Indications: useful for patients with PDN and other polyneuropathies

Precautions: concomitant use of tramadol, cardiac disease, withdrawal syndrome with abrupt discontinuation

Calcium channel alpha 2-sigma ligand anticonvulsants include the following:

■ **Gabapentin (Neurontin)**

Dosage: 100–300 mg by mouth at bedtime or 100–300 mg by mouth three times daily. Increase by 100–300 mg three times daily every 1–7 days as tolerated to a maximum of 3,600 mg daily (1,200 mg three times per day)

Caution: reduce dose for patients with impaired renal function

Precautions: renal insufficiency

■ **Pregabalin (Lyrica)**

Dosage: 50 mg by mouth three times per day or 75 mg twice per day. Increase to 300 mg daily after 3–7 days, then by 150 mg per day every 3–7 days as tolerated to a maximum of 600 mg daily

Caution: reduce dose for patients with renal impairment

Action: decreases the release of the pain-promoting substances of glutamate, norepinephrine, and substance P

Indications: useful for treatment of PHN, PDN, phantom limb pain, peripheral neuropathic pain conditions, neuropathic cancer pain, and acute and chronic spinal cord pain

Precautions: renal insufficiency

■ *Topical lidocaine (5% lidocaine patch)*

Dosage: maximum of 3 patches applied topically for a maximum of 12 hours

Indications: useful for allodynia and localized neuropathies; can be used for peripheral neuropathic pain conditions but not centrally mediated conditions

Precautions: none

Second-Line Medications
Opioids and Tramadol

The use of opioids for neuropathic pain has been discussed frequently with very little consensus. The guideline indicates the use of opioids and tramadol for neuropathic pain is indicated for:

■ Titration of a first-line medication to an efficacious dosage for prompt pain relief
■ Episodic exacerbations of severe pain
■ Acute neuropathic pain
■ Neuropathic cancer pain

Third-Line Medications

Third-line medications include antiepileptic drugs, antidepressant drugs, mexiletine, N-methyl-D-aspartate, receptor antagonists, and topical capsaicin. Because there is no strong support for use of these medications in the research literature, there is the potential for using these medications when other first- and second-line medications have failed or the patient's history indicates there is a potential for use.

Despite everyone's best efforts, the number of patients needed to treat before one patient experiences 50% improvement in pain is between 2.5 and 4 (Irving, 2005). Treating neuropathic pain can be a trial-and-error methodology. Using the recommendations of standardized guidelines can help ensure a better outcome for both the health care provider and the patient.

Randy is a patient normally seen in the primary care clinic. He has diabetes and has recently been diagnosed with cancer for which he is undergoing chemotherapy. He recently came in for his appointment and started to describe a new pain in his feet that was much worse and ached liked a toothache. He said his feet were numb and many times he could not tell he had injured a foot, and needed to be very careful so as not to hurt himself. His hands were starting to have a painful pins and needles pain that seemed to be getting worse.

When you see Randy, he tells you the pain in his feet is 8/10 and the pain in his hands is a 6/10. His sleep is being disrupted because of the pain, and none of the pain medications he has been given are helping the pain. When you ask him what medications he has been taking, he tells you Vicodin and Ambien for sleep. He says he hates to think about it, but his pain seems to be much worse since he started his chemotherapy. You suspect that Randy has a PDN that has been exacerbated by the use of vinca alkaloid chemotherapeutic drugs. What can you suggest to help Randy's pain?

Questions to Consider

1. What are the specific indications that Randy has a neuro-pathic pain?
2. Are the medications that Randy is taking the correct regimen for his pain. If not, what alternatives would there be?
3. Because Randy has PDN and chemotherapy-induced neu-ropathies, what actions could be taken to reduce the pain?
4. Will the chemotherapy-induced pain resolve once treatment is finished or the dose is decreased?
5. If Randy needs surgery for his cancer, will his surgical pain be higher than that of a patient who does not have natu-ropathic pain?

REFERENCES

Closs, S. J., Staples, V., Reid, I., Bennett, M. I., & Briggs, M. (2007). Man-aging the symptoms of neuropathic pain: An exploration of patients' experiences. *Journal of Pain & Symptom Management, 34*(4), 422–433.

Dworkin, R. H., Turk, D. C., Revicki, D. A., Harding, G., Coyne, K. S., Peirce-Sandner, S., …. Melzack, R. (2009). Development and initial validation of an expanded version of the short-form McGill pain ques-tionnaire (SF-MPQ-2). *Pain, 144*(1–2), 35–42.

Irving, G. A. (2005). Contemporary assessment and management of neu-ropathic pain. *Neurology, 64*(12), S21–S27.

Jensen, M. P., Chodroff, M. J., & Dworkin, R. H. (2007). The impact of neuropathic pain on health-related quality of life: Review and impli-cations. *Neurology, 68*(15), 1178–1182.

Polomano, R. C., & Farrar, J. T. (2006). Pain and neuropathy in cancer survivors: Surgery, radiation, and chemotherapy can cause pain. Re-search could improve its detection and treatment. *American Journal of Nursing, 106*(Suppl. 3), 39–47.

Staats, P., Argoff, C., Brewer, R., D'Arcy, Y., Gallagher, R., McCarberg, B., . . . Reisner, L. (2004). Neuropathic pain: Incorporating new con-sensus guidelines into the reality of clinical practice. *Advanced Studies in Medicine, 4*(78). Retrieved from www.JHASIM.com

ADDITIONAL RESOURCES

Dworkin, R. H., Corbin, A. E., Young, J. P., Jr., Sharma, U., LaMoreaux, M., Bockbrader, H., . . . Poole, R. (2003). Pregabalin for the treatment of postherpetic neuralgia: A randomized, placebo-controlled trial. *Neurology, 60*, 1274–1283.

16

Peripheral Neuropathic Pain Syndromes

OVERVIEW

Peripheral neuropathic pain syndromes are those conditions in which the nerves of the peripheral system are in some way damaged. This damage could be the result of an injury, surgery, a chronic illness, or an infection. Examples of these types of pain syndromes include painful diabetic neuropathy (PDN), postherpetic neuralgia (PHN), chemotherapy-related neuropathies, postthoracotomy pain syndrome (PTPS), postmastectomy pain syndrome (PMPS), phantom limb pain, or human immunodeficiency virus (HIV) neuropathy. In this chapter, the most common pain syndromes with a peripheral nerve origin will be discussed.

For most of the conditions described in Chapter 15, the use of the stepwise treatment recommendations as described in Chapter 15 are recommended. Some of the conditions have high levels of pain that often do not fully respond to opioids. Older, opioid-naïve patients often have difficulty tolerating high doses of opioids. The use of coanalgesics and topical agents combined in a multimodal plan of care are recommended. If there are specific treatment options that have been developed for a specific condition, they will be included in the appropriate section.

PERIPHERAL NEUROPATHIC PAIN SYNDROMES
AS A RESULT OF INFECTION

Postherpetic Neuralgia

The pain from PHN is one of the most intense types of pain that can be experienced with neuropathic syndromes. Patients report that the pain intensity is high, and many patients become highly sensitized to touch (allodynia), so anything coming into contact with the area of the healed infection causes extreme pain.

The cause of PHN is an infection of herpes zoster (HZ), commonly called shingles. There are an estimated 1 million episodes annually in the United States. The varicella zoster virus (chickenpox) that causes HZ can lay dormant on the dorsal root ganglia nerve endings for years and become activated much later in life or when the patient's immune system becomes compromised. The syndrome affects those patients older than 50 years when the varicella virus becomes reactivated in a specific dermatome, where a unilateral localized vesicular rash appears on only one side of the body. The rash can last for 7–10 days, and a thoracic presentation is common. There is no gender preference, but it does occur less frequently in patients with darker skin. Although it is rare, HZ can occur without any rash at all, and patients will present with a localized severe pain in the area of the affected dermatome.

PHN is common after HZ infection, with about 10% to 18% of the HZ patients developing PHN. After the healing of the vesicles, the affected area can become highly sensitized so that even the mild touch of clothing in the area is extremely painful. The sensitivity in the healed area is caused by unprovoked, spontaneous neuronal firing and a lowered neuronal activation threshold (Khaliq, Alam, & Puri, 2008). Thermal hyperalgesia is also very characteristic of PHN.

Patients describe the pain of PHN as burning, painful numbness or tingling, electric shocklike pain, or incredibly painful itching (Morantz & Torrey, 2005). If the herpes eruption was on a dermatome located on the face, there may be vision, hearing, or oral effects. The pain from PHN can occur from 1 to 6 months after the onset of the vesicular eruption. It is described as severe in intensity and can interfere with sleep, affect the ability to perform activities of daily life, and decrease appetite. Patients may also feel as if they have an untreatable condition because the pain is not often relieved by normal medications for pain. Unfortunately, the pain of PHN may persist for weeks, months, or years.

Which patients who have a HZ outbreak will develop PHN? There are some risk factors that can help pinpoint the most likely candidates for PHN. These include:

- A prodromal pain in the area prior to the rash outbreak
- High levels of pain with the original HZ outbreak (Hampton, 2005)
- Older age at onset
- More psychosocial interference in role, social, and physical functioning; personality disorders
- Compromised immune functions (Katz et al., 2005)

To minimize the possibility of PHN, patients with HZ should take antiviral treatment at the onset of the eruption. With no antiviral treatment, 40% of the patients with HZ will develop PHN, although the incidence drops to 20% in those patients who take the antiviral medications (Hampton, 2005). After many years in development, a new HZ vaccine has been released for patients who are older and at greater risk for HZ and PHN. This new development will hopefully decrease the cases of HZ and subsequently decrease the cases of PHN.

The 5% lidocaine patch (Lidoderm) was developed for use in this condition. It is a prescription strength topical local anesthetic application in patch form that penetrates deeper into the dermis to provide a local anesthetic effect in the area of PHN. The newest medication that is considered for this condition is the Quetensa 8% capsaicin patch. It is a patch with high concentrations of capsaicin cream that requires a health care provider to place it for a 60-minute treatment. Prior to the treatment, the area needs to be treated with a topical anesthetic agent, such as a eutectic mixture of local anesthetic, so the patient will be able to tolerate the treatment. There is emerging evidence for the use of combination treatments for PHN. Interventional options, such as epidural steroid injections, trigger point injections, or acupuncture, have limited evidence for use but have anecdotal reports of efficacy.

> | *Clinical* | If the affected area is along the trigeminal nerve distribution |
> | *Pearl* | the patient should be sent to an ophthalmologist for evaluation |
> | | of visual effects. |

HIV-ASSOCIATED SENSORY NEUROPATHY

HIV-associated sensory neuropathy (HIV-SN) is a result of damage to the peripheral nervous system caused by the HIV infection and is most often located in the feet. Patients who have HIV-SN report pain that is aching, painful numbness, or burning. Hyperalgesia and allodynia are common (Abrams et al., 2007).

Although the condition responds to most usual drug therapies, a unique approach was trialed in a group of 50 patients with HIV-SN. The average daily pain score for the patients was at least three on the Numeric Rating Scale. Patients who had previously indicated that they had use cannabis at least six times in their lives were assigned to smoke cannabis cigarettes. The first cannabis cigarette reduced daily pain scores by a median of 72% versus 15% for the placebo group. Overall, the study participants who smoked cannabis reduced daily pain by 34% (Abrams et al., 2007).

Although this study had the patients actually smoke a cannabis cigarette, there are drugs currently in the development stage that have the active ingredients of cannabis but do not produce euphoria. Because neuropathic pain is so difficult to treat, researchers are continually looking for options that are worth developing for treating this type of pain. Although this cannabis study proves the effect of the drug, using a legal and equally effective medication designed for this specific treatment, such as the new cannabis derivatives, will provide another alternative for treatment.

PERIPHERAL NEUROPATHIC PAIN AS A RESULT OF NERVE ENTRAPMENT SYNDROMES OR POSTOPERATIVE PAIN SYNDROMES

Postmastectomy Pain Syndrome

Women who undergo lumpectomy or mastectomy are at risk for developing postmastectomy pain syndrome (PMPS), a neuropathic syndrome affecting the chest wall, axilla, or medial aspect of the surgical arm. About 20% of the women who undergo mastectomy or lumpectomy with axillary node dissection develop PMPS (Palomano & Farrar, 2006). The condition is more common in younger women and those who are overweight (Palomano & Farrar, 2006).

The syndrome can also include a phantom breast syndrome if a patient has had a mastectomy. In this presentation, the patient feels like the surgically removed breast is still present and pain can be experienced in much the same way a patient who has had a limb amputated can still feel pain in the amputated extremity.

PMPS is a direct result of surgically created nerve damage during lumpectomy or mastectomy that results in a neuropathic pain syndrome. Because the condition is associated with breast cancer, the continuing pain after surgery is often overlooked in favor of the ongoing treatment of the disease. The patients may also be unwilling to talk about strange sensations, painful pins and needles, or painful numbness that is occurring on the surgical side of the chest or the surgical side axilla, fearing they will be told that it is not a "real" pain. The intensity of the pain can limit rehabilitation or a return to full activity after surgery. The patient may report difficulty raising the arm or participating in physical therapy to restore function to the arm on the surgical side. Other pain complaints that patients have reported are general aching and burning in the surgical site and the axilla and medial aspect of the affected area, and paroxysmal episodes of shooting and lancinating pain (Wallace & Wallace, 1997).

Because PMPS can limit the movement of the affected shoulder and arm, it is important to intervene early in the syndrome to help the patients prevent any functional limitations that can occur as the result of disuse. It is also important to believe the patients report of pain so that adequate treatment for the pain can be provided, and the patient can continue with rehabilitation of the affected arm and shoulder. Providing coanalgesic medications, such as antidepressants, can help reduce the pain intensity and promote participation in rehabilitation.

Postthoracotomy Pain Syndrome

When patients undergo a thoracotomy, the intercostal nerves located along the ribs are at risk for damage and impingement. When the intercostal nerves are damaged or compressed during surgery, the patient can develop PTPS (Wallace & Wallace, 1997). About 50% to 80% of patients who have had a thoracotomy continue to experience chronic pain in the area of the surgery (Palomano & Farrar, 2006).

About 5% of the patients who have chronic pain will develop long-term debilitating pain with a neuropathic component (Palomano & Farrar, 2006). The pain of PTPS can be very severe in nature. Patients have described this pain as "feeling as if a blow torch is being run back and forth over my chest" or dysesthetic with episodes of shooting pain. Allodynia is also common in the painful area (Wallace & Wallace, 1997).

With both PMPS and PTPS, the area of the scar can also be highly sensitive and painful. Some patients describe this pain as itchiness (Wallace & Wallace, 1997). There are some effective treatments for these two conditions, and the treatment options can be found in Chapter 15.

Phantom Limb Syndrome

When a limb is amputated, especially a lower extremity, the patient is at risk for a neuropathic pain called *phantom limb syndrome.* Patients may feel the amputated limb is still there and feel pain in the amputated extremity as if it were still attached to the body. About 30% to 80% of all patients who undergo amputation of a limb, either leg or arm, will experience phantom limb pain (Eichenberger et al., 2008).

With this syndrome, the patient will report feeling the leg even though they can look at their body and know it has been removed. Some patients feel as if the limb has been "frozen" into a certain position that may be related to the position of limb prior to amputation.

Characteristics of phantom limb pain include:

- Onset within the first few days of amputation
- Intermittent rather than constant
- Pain coming from the part of the amputated extremity farthest from the body, such as the foot of a leg
- Has been described as shooting, stabbing, boring, squeezing, throbbing, or burning
- May be triggered be weather changes, or pressure on the remaining portion of the limb (http://www.mayoclinic.com, retrieved July 2009)

After the amputation, the nerves serving the amputated limb rewire themselves, which may the source of some of the strange feelings or pain. Patients may also report that they feel the foot coming closer to their body. This telescoping effect is also believed to be the result of neuronal remodeling after surgery. The effect can be unsettling to the patient, and they need reassurance that the feeling will gradually resolve after the nerves have completed their neuronal remodeling.

In a study of 20 postamputation patients with phantom limb pain, a trial of calcitonin and ketamine to reduce the pain was conducted using a double-blind placebo-controlled design. Because the two drugs are classed as N-methyl-D-aspartate (NMDA) antagonists, the research team was attempting to aim the process at the point in the pain cascade where NMDA receptors were activated. Findings demonstrated that ketamine alone could reduce the phantom limb pain, but calcitonin alone did not (Eichenberger et al., 2008). Combining the medications did not reduce pain. Given the lack of response to the pain threshold portion of the study, the research team indicated that peripheral mechanisms are unlikely to be the source of phantom limb pain (Eichenberger et al., 2008).

NEUROPATHIC PAIN AS A RESULT OF CHRONIC ILLNESS

Painful Diabetic Neuropathy

Diabetes is very common in the United States. Estimates are that diabetes affects about 17 million people of all ages in the United States. The incidence of PDN is estimated to be 37% to 45% of patients with type 2 diabetes and 54% to 59% of patients with type 1 diabetes (Wernicke et al., 2006).

PDN is exacerbated by poorly controlled blood sugar levels and occurs as a stocking glove-like distribution most commonly affecting the feet. Patients who have PDN report allodynia and pain that is sharp, stabbing, painful numbness in the feet, and burning pain in the feet. The intensity of pain increases at night. Some patients have reported that PDN is like walking on broken glass, with sharp pricking and stinging sensations in the feet. Patients have also reported a lack of proprioception for their feet, creating an inability to locate their feet in space. This can make injury very common because the patient stubs toes and runs into furniture that they cannot feel. All diabetics should be taught to inspect their feet nightly for injury or rubbed spots from shoes that they may not realize are rubbing against toes.

There are a variety of medications that can be used to treat PDN. The selective serotonin norepinephrine reuptake inhibitor (SSNRI) medications duloxetine and pregabalin are two medications that have Federal Drug Administration (FDA) approval for treating PDN. Unfortunately, only 42% of patients taking medication for PDN indicated they were satisfied with their current treatment options.

NEUROPATHIC PAIN AS A RESULT OF TREATMENTS

Chemotherapy-Related Neuropathies

Patients with cancer who take chemotherapy as a treatment for their disease can develop neuropathies that develop in a stocking glove distribution. The treatment is aimed at curing the cancer, but the neuropathy that develops as a result of the treatment can be very painful. Chemotherapy drugs that can cause these neuropathies include:

- Vinca alkaloids
- Taxanes
- Platinum-based compounds
- Cytosine arabinoside
- fluorouracil and antimitotics (Palomano & Farrar, 2006)

Because the drugs that cause these neuropathies are being used to fight cancer, the adverse effect of the neuropathies is highly unfortunate. It is difficult to estimate prevalence of the condition because each patient has different and confounding factors, such as renal clearance, alcohol use, genetic susceptibility, and so forth, that all play an individual role in producing neuropathies (Palomano & Farrar, 2006).

Chemotherapy-related neuropathies can produce a variety of symptoms that can include:

- Loss of sensation
- Pain
- Motor dysfunction (e.g., foot drop)
- Numbness
- Tingling
- Other painful dysesthesia or paresthesia (Palomano & Farrar, 2006)

The neuropathies typically affect the hands and feet. The onset of symptoms can be very swift—30 to 60 minutes after the infusion with oxaliplatin—but patients receiving Cisplatin can develop symptoms in approximately 30 days after starting the infusions (Palomano & Farrar, 2006).

Dose reduction can be effective in controlling the neuropathy but, because the drugs are being used to treat a life-threatening illness, this may not always be the best option. There are medications, such as antidepressants, anticonvulsants, and topical agents, that can be used to treat the neuropathies once they occur. Although there are some patients who report that the chemotherapy-related neuropathies improve after treatment, there are also some patients who report continued neuropathies years after treatment has been completed.

SUMMARY

This chapter provides an overview of neuropathic pain and pain syndromes that have their origin in the peripheral nervous system. The following chapter will discuss pain syndromes that have their origin in the central nervous system.

Marcella Smith is a 72-year-old widow who has been referred to the pain clinic for treatment of pain related to PHN. She had a case of HZ (shingles) 6 months ago and continues to have a significant pain that she rates as 6 out of 10. She has tried a variety of medications that have provided only moderate relief. Her primary care provider has sent her to the pain clinic, hoping to find a solution to the pain. When you meet Marcella, she tells you, "This has been a horrible year. I had shingles right after Christmas and the pain was terrible. The burning was unbelievable. I thought it would get better once the rash healed, but it didn't. I still can't have clothing over that area touch my body. I wear housecoats mainly. The pain medication helps some, but I can't sleep very well. I have to take a sleeping pill. Any pressure on my chest area just starts the pain right up. Is there some kind of treatment or medication that will help the pain."

Current medications:
Gabapentin 300 mg by mouth three times per day
Ambien 10 mg by mouth at bedtime daily
Vicodin 1 tablet by mouth every 4 hours as needed pain

Questions to Consider

1. Would you recommend opioids to treat this pain?
2. What type of topical medication could help Marcella's pain?
3. What indicator was a hint that Marcella's pain would progress to PHN?
4. Would a trigger point injection be helpful for this pain?
5. Will it be possible to get this pain to a tolerable level eventually?

REFERENCES

Abrams, D. I., Jay, C. A., Shade, S. B., Vizoso, H., Reda, H., Press, S., . . . Peterson, K. L. (2007). Cannabis in painful HIV-associated sensory neuropathy: A randomized placebo-controlled trial. *Neurology, 68*(7), 515–521.

Eichenberger, U., Neff, F., Sveticic, G., Bjorgo, S., Petersen-Feklix, S., Arendt-Neilsen, L., & Curatolo, M. (2008). Chronic phantom limb pain: The effects of calcitonin, ketamine, and their combination on pain and sensory thresholds. *Anesthesia & Analgesia, 106*(4), 1265–1273.

Hampton, T. (2005). When shingles wanes but the pain does not: Researchers target chronic postherpetic neuralgia. *JAMA, 293*(20), 2459–2460.

Katz, J., McDermott, M. P., Cooper, E. M., Walther, R. R., Sweeney, E. W., & Dworkin, R. H. (2005). Psychosocial risk factors for postherpetic neuralgia: A prospective study of patients with herpes zoster. *The Journal of Pain, 6*(12), 782–790.

Khaliq, W., Alam, S., & Puri, N. (2007). Topical lidocaine for the treatment of postherpetic neuralgia. *The Cochrane Database of Systematic Reviews,* (2).

Morantz, C., & Torrey, B. (2005). Practice guideline briefs. *American Family Physician, 71*(4), 1–3.

Palomano, R. C., & Farrar, J. T. (2006). Pain and neuropathy in cancer survivors. Surgery, radiation, and chemotherapy can cause pain; Research could improve its detection and treatment. *American Journal of Nursing, 106*(Suppl. 3), 39–47.

Wallace, A., & Wallace, M. (1997). Postmastectomy and postthoracotomy pain. *Anesthesiology Clinics of North America, 15*(2), 353–370.

Wernicke, J. F., Prichett, Y. L., D'Souza, D. N., Waniger, A., Tran, P., Iyenger, S., & Raskin, J. (2006). A randomized controlled trial of duloxetine in diabetic peripheral neuropathic pain. *Neurology, 67*(8), 1411–1420.

ADDITIONAL RESOURCES

Closs, S. J., Staples, V., Reid, I., Bennet, M. I., & Briggs, M. (2007). Managing the symptoms of neuropathic pain: An exploration of patients' experiences. *Journal of Pain & Symptom Management, 34*(4), 422–433.

D'Arcy, Y. (2006). Postmastectomy pain syndrome and other difficult to treat neuropathic pain syndromes: An overview. *The Pain Practitioner, 16*(2), 41–49.

Dworkin, R. H., Corbin, A. E., Young, J. P., Jr., Sharma, U., LaMoreaux, L., Bockbader, H., . . . Poole, R. M. (2003). Pregabalin for the treatment of postherpetic neuralgia: A randomized, placebo-controlled trial. *Neurology, 60*, 1274–1283.

Irving, G. (2005). Contemporary assessment and management of neuropathic pain. *Neurology, 64*(12), S21–S27.

Jensen, M. P., Chodroff, M. J., & Dworkin, R. H. (2007). The impact of neuropathic pain on health-related quality of life: Review and implications. *Neurology, 68*(15), 1178–1182.

Staats, P., Argoff, C., Brewer, R., D'Arcy, Y., Gallagher, R., McCarberg, B., et al. (2004). Neuropathic pain: Incorporating new consensus guidelines into the reality of clinical practice. *Advanced Studies in Medicine, 4*(78).

17

Central Pain Syndromes

OVERVIEW

Neuropathic pain that has a centrally mediated origin and is defined as "pain associated with lesions of the central nervous system" (Nicholson, 2004). It involves the spinal nerves, postsynaptic junction with the peripheral nervous system, spinal cord, brain (the thalamus has been implicated in some of the central pain syndromes), and cerebral cortex. It is one of the most difficult pain complaints to treat because the source mechanisms are so complex, and many are not fully understood.

What we do know about centrally mediated syndromes is that continued painful stimuli can cause activation and recruitment of additional pain, causing substances and mechanisms such a neuronal plasticity, activation of the N-methyl-D-aspartate (NMDA) system, and the "wind-up" phenomenon. These neuronal changes are second stage pain-promoting mechanisms that can increase pain intensity; once they are activated, they are difficult to deactivate.

Centrally mediated syndromes are also related to the activation of the peripheral nervous system and chemical responses. With repeated pain stimuli, peripheral and central nerves become increasingly sensitized and hyperexcited through increased sodium channel activity, producing conditions such as allodynia. Once the pain is being produced by a central mechanism, it does not require peripheral input to continue producing pain. Centrally mediated pain is a self-generating phenomenon that is a vicious circle of self-promotion without any inhibitory mechanism.

Some common types of central pain syndromes include the following:

- Poststroke pain
- Complex regional pain syndrome (CRPS) type I and type II
- Spinal cord injury pain
- Multiple sclerosis pain
- Possible fibromyalgia

When the patient talks about his or her neuropathic pain, he or she may have very different symptoms, such as odd dysesthetic sensations, pain sensations that are hard to locate, or descriptors that are hard to define, such as "waves of fire rising over my body periodically." There can also be a variation in the consistency of the pain presentation, which makes treating the condition all the more difficult. Consequently, this type of pain is often diagnosed incorrectly or treated with medications that may not relieve the symptoms. It can be very challenging for the health care provider to attempt to control such poorly defined and generalized pain.

In addition, the pain intensity can be very severe and vary in intensity at different periods during the day. Because the pain is so significant, it can affect the quality of life for patients and cause a major impact on their functionality, sleep, emotional lives, and social relationships.

The effect on the functioning and quality of life in patients with neuropathic pain can be quite substantial. In a study of both peripheral and central neuropathic pain patients, there were negative effects reported in the domains of physical functioning, emotional role, and social functioning (Jensen, Chodroff, & Dworkin, 2007). Important impairments were seen with sleep, physical functioning, and emotional functioning (Jensen, Chodroff, & Dworkin, 2007). Although the data suggest that there are some very basic impairments on individual areas of the patients' lives, in the assessment of the global quality of life, the research identified the fact that the higher the pain intensity, the lower the level of global quality of life (Jensen, Chodroff, & Dworkin, 2007).

It is understandable that patients with these syndromes would become depressed and feel that they have little control over the condition. To avoid overlooking important quality of life or psychosocial issues, such as anxiety or depression, patients should be assessed for these conditions at every clinic visit. Patients may be able to cope much better with the chronic pain if depression is addressed and treated.

CAUSES OF CENTRAL NEUROPATHIC PAIN

Neuropathic pain that has a central origin is caused by a lesion or dysfunction in one or more of the structures in the central nervous system. Central pain can be divided into two broad categories: spinal-cord–related pain or brain-related pain (Nicholson, 2004).

Spinal-cord–related central pain is most often caused by some form of trauma. The most common type of trauma is motor vehicle accidents, which account for 60% to 70% of all trauma-related spinal cord pain (Nicholson, 2004). Other less common causes of spinal cord central pain include the following:

■ Congenital disease
■ Inflammation
■ Neoplasm
■ Iatrogenic cause (related to surgery)
■ Vascular disease (Nicholson, 2004)

Brain-related central pain can be caused by events such as stroke. In stroke, the brain receives an insult, such as a clot or an infarct, that causes brain tissue death and tissue swelling. Of the 700,000 Americans who experience stroke, about 8% of the patients develop central-poststroke pain (CPSP). This centrally mediated pain syndrome can present differently in patients affected by the condition. Some patients complain of a burning sensation, whereas others complain of allodynia.

Exhibit 17.1

MD HAS CP

Muscle pains: cramping, bandlike constriction, crushing sensations
Dysesthesias: abnormal, unpleasant, poorly localized sensations
Hyperpathia: heightened response to noxious stimuli
Allodynia: a nonpainful stimulus, such as touch, becomes painful
Shooting/lancinating pain: intermittent pain that is easy to localize
Circulatory pain: pain described as pins and needles, stings, jabs, or walking on broken glass
Peristaltic/visceral pain: pain described as bloating, bladder fullness, or burning with urination

Source: From Nicholson, 2004.

In the brain, the thalamus is thought to be the source of CPSP. Although this type of injury affects motor pathways, it has also been suggested that somatosensory pathways sustain damage that can manifest as long as 1 to 6 years after the main event (Nicholson, 2004).

There are certain characteristic symptoms with central neuropathic pain syndromes such as stroke. These can be explained the use of the acronym "MD HAS CP" (Exhibit 17.1).

CENTRAL PAIN SYNDROMES

Poststroke Pain

CPSP occurs in a small number of stroke patients (about 8% of the stroke patient population). It may occur within 1–2 months after the initial stroke, but it can also manifest at 1–6 years (Kumar et al., 2009; Nicholson, 2004). It is not one of the most frequent complaints that stroke patients have, so it may be overlooked for a period of time before it is identified and diagnosed.

The three proposed mechanisms for CPSP are the following:

- Central sensitization
- Imbalance of stimuli
- Central disinhibition (Kumar et al., 2009)

The pain is most commonly thought to originate in the thalamus (Kumar et al., 2009). Central sensitization can occur when nerve damage release excitatory neurotransmitters and neuropeptides, such as glutamate, calcitonin gene-related peptide, and substance P. This release can also cause excitatory toxicity of inhibitory neurons (Irving, 2005). This means that once the pain starts and is established, the mechanisms designed to stop the pain may be disengaged.

One of the biggest problems with CPSP is that it has a wide variation in presentation, but it can interfere with rehabilitation. CPSP can be either evoked or spontaneous (Kumar et al., 2009). If the pain is spontaneous, the patient may complain of the following:

- Aching or squeezing
- Burning
- Pricking or lacerating
- Shooting or throbbing
- Heaviness or a cold feeling (Kumar et al., 2009)

If the pain is evoked, it may stimulate allodynia or hyperalgesia, and the patient may complain of the following:

- There may be a punctate type pain or a thermally induced pain response to heat and/or cold.
- This type of pain may be steady or it may be dynamic and increase at certain periods of time (Kumar et al., 2009).

No matter what type of descriptor or complaint, the patients will experience hemibody pain on the side of the body contralateral to the stroke. The areas of the body that are most often affected by CPSP are the trunk, arm, leg, or face (Kumar et al., 2009).

The recommended first-line treatment options for CPSP are the following:

- amitriptyline
- lamotrigine (Kumar et al., 2009; Nicholson, 2004)

Second-line treatment options include the following:

- fluvoxamine
- gabapentin
- mexiletine

One controversial nondrug treatment for CPSP is deep brain stimulation (DBS). DBS has been found to be effective for patients who have had a thalamic type of stroke (Nicholson, 2004), but it may not work for every patient with CPSP (Kumar et al., 2009). Repetitive transcranial magnetic stimulation has been used to treat CPSP of the face, legs, and arms. It has proved effective for pain relief, and the treatments have maintained the pain relief for 2 weeks after the last session (Kumar et al., 2009).

Patient selection for this type of treatment should be done very carefully and limited to those patients who are pharmacoresistent. Because efficacy is not established, these advanced interventional techniques should be reserved for those patients who have resistant pain and for whom there is the possibility of a positive outcome. These options are designed as last-line therapies that are used when all other options have been partially effective or ineffective.

Complex Regional Pain Syndrome

CRPS types I and II were historically called *causalgia*. Causalgia is a burning pain associated with trophic skin changes due to peripheral nerve damage. It has been reported in medical practices since the mid-1800s (Harden, 2005). At that time, it was felt that a dysregulation of the sympathetic nervous system was the cause of the pain. During the Civil War, the use of ammunition such as "minie balls" that caused a great deal of tissue damage were said to account for the development of what was then classed as causalgia in war veterans (Harden, 2005).

Because the belief was that this type of pain was caused by the sympathetic nervous system, most efforts at treatment were aimed at trying to affect the sympathetic nervous system. Sympathectomies using alcohol or phenol injections were used to temporarily or permanently interrupt the sympathetic nervous system. Surgical ablation was also performed for the same purpose. Unfortunately, evidence has shown that these procedures had as many poor outcomes as positive, and there is no recommendation for use (Cepeda, 2005). Because the evidence is weak for this practice, more research on this technique is indicated. Adverse effects from these procedures include the following:

- Worsening pain
- Creating a new pain syndrome
- Abnormal forms of sweating, such as hyperhidrosis (Mailis-Gagnon & Furlan, 2009)

Because of the association with the sympathetic nervous system, the pain condition known as causalgia was renamed *reflex sympathetic dystrophy* and more recently complex regional pain syndrome I & II. Patients who are at risk for the syndrome now known as CRPS are those who have sustained an acute tissue injury, such as a crush injury, or have had repeated tissue trauma, such as repeated surgical procedures for carpal tunnel syndrome, for example. These patients will report continued high levels of pain intensity, with little relief when standard pain relief options are used. This lack of pain relief can be attributed to another facet of this syndrome: reduced endogenous pain inhibition (Edwards, 2005). CRPS is most commonly found in upper or lower extremities. Any acute pain patient who continues to report high levels of pain should be evaluated for CRPS.

Clinical Pearl	There are two types of CRPS, as follows: ■ CRPS I corresponds to the International Association for the Study of Pain (IASP) criteria for CRPS and does not require the presence of a nerve lesion. ■ CRPS II incorporates all of the criteria for CRPS I but includes the presence of a nerve lesion.

The IASP has developed criteria for diagnosing CRPS, which include the following:

- Initiating noxious event
- Continuing pain
- Allodynia or hyperalgesia where the pain is disproportionate to the precipitating event
- Evidence (at sometime) of edema
- Changes in skin blood flow
- Abnormal sudomotor activity in the affected area (Harden, 2005)

Other symptoms that are common in patients who have CRPS include the following:

- Changes in temperature when compared with the unaffected extremity (80% develop)
- Extreme sensitivity to temperature changes (e.g., cold, heat)
- Changes in hair and nail growth
- Weakness and tremor (Harden, 2005)

The real cause of CRPS is unknown but is thought to be linked to one of three mechanisms:

- Enhanced peripheral neurogenic inflammation
- Dysfunction of the sympathetic nervous system
- Structural reorganization in the central nervous system (Fechir, Geber, & Birklein, 2008)

There is some current research to determine if there is any causative connection between CRPS and an immune system action in which autoantibodies are allowed to attack nervous system structures (Blaes et al., 2004).

No matter what the cause, the pain that a patient with CRPS reports is severe and long lasting, and in most cases does not respond well to medications. The average age of a CRPS patient ranges from 36 to 46 years; the syndrome is more commonly found in women (Ghai & Dureja, 2004). These are patients who are most often employed and are in the most productive years of their lives. The condition can have a significant negative effect on the quality of life and functionality of these patients.

The pain may become so severe that patients will not use the affected extremity. This can lead to chronic disuse and in the most severe cases contractures, which can become permanent. Treatment options provide suboptimal relief, with only 29% of the patients in a retrospective study reporting they were pain free, whereas 64% of the patients reported severe level pain, with an average daily pain rating of 7 on the Numeric Rating Scale (Ghai & Dureja, 2004).

Treating CRPS-related pain requires a multimodal approach using medications, regional anesthesia techniques such as blocks, and aggressive physical therapy to retain function. Desensitization and edema reduction are early treatments in any therapy program. The earlier the condition is diagnosed and interventions initiated, the better the final outcome will be. The use of interventional techniques, such as blocks or epidural and intrathecal catheters with local anesthetic alone or combined with ketamine, allows for manipulation of the extremity with the least possible pain (Ghai & Dureja, 2004).

The goal of treatment is to allow the patients to engage in the fullest possible rehabilitation of the affected extremity. Harden (2005) recommends the following types of treatments for the symptoms of CRPS. For pain at lower levels, use analgesics and regional techniques such as blocks; for higher levels of pain, consider opioids and more advanced regional techniques such as implanted epidural catheters. For pain syndromes that are more difficult to treat, use anticonvulsants, NMDA antagonists, or sodium channel blockers. Inflammation is responsive to steroids and NSAIDs (see Chapter 3). Severe vasomotor symptoms may respond to nifedipine or blocks.

No matter what treatment is selected, the overall goal is to restore maximum functionality, which requires intensive and long-term physical therapy, combined with the most effective treatment strategies.

Multiple Sclerosis

Multiple sclerosis (MS) is an autoimmune disease that causes demyelination of nerves. There are about 400,000 people in the United States who have been diagnosed with MS, of which 42% to 65% complain of pain (Rog et al., 2009). Most patients who have pain with this chronic illness can be managed with over-the-counter analgesics, such as acetaminophen, or a short course of nonsteroidal anti-inflammatory drugs (NSAIDs). However, there are a number of patients who have pain that is refractory to most common treatments.

The pain that patients with MS complain of is in many cases a mixed presentation of acute, paroxysmal, and chronic pain (Rog et al., 2009). The pain occurs most commonly in the lower extremities and is bilateral (Rog et al.). Because pain is not the focus of treatment for MS, the pain complaint may be overlooked. A secondary condition that may accompany the pain of MS is trigeminal neuralgia, which is pain across the face along the dermatome served by the trigeminal nerves. The presence of trigeminal neuralgia in a patient with MS may indicate brain stem demyelination and is also considered to be centrally induced (Rog et al., 2009).

As with other chronic pain conditions, medication may produce a variety of side effects that may be difficult to tolerate. A Cochrane Review is underway to assess effectiveness and tolerability of medications that can be used to treat the central pain syndromes of MS.

SUMMARY

Centrally mediated pain syndromes are some of the most difficult to diagnose and treat. The primary care practitioner may spend many visits trying to determine what the cause of the pain is, and it takes trial and error to find the right medication combinations and dose.

This area of pain medicine is continually evolving. Most recently, it has been determined that fibromyalgia pain is a result of central amplification where the pain stimulus is augmented and dramatically enhanced. This makes even a hug painful. In addition to these new findings, there is an indication that the mu receptor sites in these patients are fully occupied, making the use of opioids a poor option for treatment. As science progresses, more and more information will be developed about centrally mediated syndromes that will lead to better treatment options and outcomes for patients.

Steve Burns, who is 16 years old, is an athlete in high school playing three different sports: basketball, football, and baseball. He also has a part-time job in a gas station that stocks a small amount of food supplies. Part of Steve's job is to stock these supplies. Six months ago, he dropped a case of bottled soda on his foot. He was seen in the emergency room and treated for a muscle strain and soft-tissue injury. The pain was surprisingly very severe, and Steve did not get good pain relief from the medications that were provided. He has not been able to play sports at school, and he uses crutches to get around. He is being sent to a pain specialist because his pain does not seem to respond to any of the medications that his primary physician has tried. He has had consults to an orthopedist, a physiatrist, a psychologist, and a physical therapist. His primary care physician does not want to continue to prescribe opioids for pain in such a young patient. He is afraid Steve will become addicted to them.

Steve tells the pain specialist, "I don't know what to do. I used to be so active, and I played a lot of sports. Now all I can do is get from home to school and back home. I can't really enjoy my life. I play video games all the time, and my schoolwork is suffering. I used to get As and Bs, but I definitely have slipped down to steady Cs.

The pain in my foot is unbelievable. It just burns and aches. I can't bear to touch it to the ground or wear shoes. It feels so achy cold all the time. I don't like taking medications, and they really don't help either. Strange as it may sound, I feel like my other foot is starting to have the same type of pain as the injured one. Is there some kind of treatment that will make this better?"

Current medications:

Vicodin 1 tablet by mouth, four times per day as needed
Ibuprofen 400 mg by mouth, three times per day
Neurontin 300 mg by mouth, three times per day

Questions to Consider

■ What kind of pain syndrome does Steve have? Can it spread to his other foot?
■ What types of medication changes would you make?
■ Will physical therapy be helpful? What might have to be done to allow Steve to participate in the activity?
■ Is there a role for topical agents? If so what kind?
■ Is an NSAID a good choice for pain relief? What risks do they have for a patient such as Steve?

REFERENCES

Blaes, F., Schmitz, K., Tschernatsch, M., Kaps, M., Krasenbrink, I., Hempelmann, G., & Bräu, M. E. (2004). Autoimmune etiology of complex regional pain syndrome (M. Sudeck). *Neurology, 63*(9), 1734–1736.

Cepeda, M. S., Carr, D. B., & Lau, J. (2005). Local anesthetic sympathetic blockade for complex regional pain syndrome. *The Cochrane Database of Systematic Reviews*, 4.

Edwards, R. R. (2005). Individual differences in endogenous pain modulation as a risk factor for chronic pain. *Neurology, 65*(3), 437–443.

Fechir, M., Geber, C., & Birklein, F. (2008). Evolving understandings about complex regional pain syndrome and its treatment. *Current Pain & Headache Reports, 12*(3), 186–191.

Ghai, B., & Dureja, G. P. (2004). Complex regional pain syndrome: A review. *Journal of Postgraduate Medicine, 50*(4), 300–307.

Harden, R. N. (2005). Pharmacotherapy of complex regional pain syndrome. *American Journal of Physical Medicine and Rehabilitation, 84*(3), S17–S28.

Jensen, M. P., Chodroff, M. J., & Dworkin, R. H. (2007). The impact of neuropathic pain on health-related quality of life: Review and implications. *Neurology, 68*(15), 1178–1182.

Kumar, B., Kalita, J., Kumar, G., & Misra, U. (2009). Central poststroke pain: A review of pathophysiology and treatment. *Anesthesia & Analgesia, 108*, 1645–1657.

Mailis-Gagnon, A., & Furlan, A. (2009). Sympathectomy for neuropathic pain. *Cochrane Database of Systematic Reviews*, 2.

Nicholson, B. D. (2004). Evaluation and treatment of central pain syndromes. *Neurology, 62*(5), S30–S36.

Rog, D., Young, C., Hollis, S., & Freide, T. (2009). Treatment of neuropathic pain for multiple sclerosis. *Cochrane Database of Systematic Reviews*, 2.

ADDITIONAL RESOURCES

Dworkin, R. H., O'Connor, A. B., Backonja, M., Farrar, J. T., Finnerup, N. B., Jensen, T. S., . . . Wallace, M. S. (2007). Pharmacologic management of neuropathic pain: Evidence-based recommendations. *Pain, 132*, 237–251.

Fishbain, D. A., Lewis, J. E., Cutler, R., Cole, B., Rosomoff, H. L., & Rosomoff, R S. (2008). Can the neuropathic pain scale discriminate between non-neuropathic and neuropathic pain? *Pain Medicine, 9*(2), 149–160.

Selected Websites for Guidelines

EVIDENCE-BASED WEBSITES

- The Cochrane Collaboration (http://www.cochrane.org) reviews and grades current scientific research. It has several pain management study groups.
- The National Guideline Clearinghouse (http://www.guideline.gov) has a large number of clinical guidelines and is support by the Agency for Healthcare Research and Quality.
- The Joanna Briggs Institute (http://www.joannabriggs.edu.au) specializes in evidence-based resources for nurses, medicine, and allied health.

PAIN SOCIETY AND DISEASE-SPECIFIC WEBSITES

- The American Chronic Pain Association (www.theacpa.org) has information of support groups for patients with chronic pain and general information on chronic pain.
- American Pain Society (www.ampainsoc.org) has information on low-back pain, cancer pain, fibromyalgia pain, acute pain, chronic opioid therapy, and pain management in primary care.
- The American Society of Anesthesiologists (www.asahq.org) hosts perioperative guidelines.
- The American Pain Foundation (www.painfoundation.org) provides help for finding general pain information.
- The American Academy of Pain Medicine (www.painmed.org) has position statements on practice issues

- The American Society for Pain Management Nursing (www.aspmn.org) supplies position statements.
- The American Society for Perioperative Nursing (www.aspan.org) provides pain, comfort, and postoperative nausea guidelines.
- The National Fibromyalgia Association (www.fmaware.org) has information on fibromyalgia pain and symptom management.
- The Oncology Nursing Society (http://www.ons.org/) has cancer pain management information
- The American Society of Regional Anesthesia (www.asra.com) provides epidural/anticoagulation position statements.
- The American Geriatrics Society (www.americangeriatrics.org) has guidelines and statements on pain in older patients.

B

Equianalgesic Conversion Table

Equianalgesic Table for Opioid Conversion

Analgesics	Generic	Brand Name	Oral dose	Parenteral	
Immediate release	Morphine	Roxanol, MSIR	30 milligrams	10 milligrams	Relative potency 1:6 with acute dosing and 1:2 to 1:3 with chronic dosing
	Oxycodone	Roxicodone, Oxy IR	20 milligrams	NA	
	Hydromorphone	Dilaudid	7.5 milligrams	1.5 milligrams	
	Oxymorphone	Opana, Numorphan	10 milligrams	1 milligram	Extended half life with short-acting oral form
	Hydrocodone	Vicodin, Lortab	30 milligrams	NA	
	Fentanyl	Sublimaze	NA	100 micrograms	
	Methadone	Dolophine	5-10 milligrams	10 milligrams	Use with caution: Half life of 12-150 hours accumulates with repeated dosing
	Meperidine	Demerol	NR	NR	Use with caution. Toxic metabolite normerperidine can cause seizures

Controlled Release	Generic	Brand Name	Oral dose	Parenteral	
Not recommended for opioid naïve patients	Morphine	MSContin, Avinza, Kadian	20-30		
	Oxycodone	Oxycontin	20-30 milligrams		
	Fentanyl transdermal	Duragesic	NA	25 micrograms	

Basic Intravenous conversion: Morphine 1 milligram = Dilaudid 0.2 milligrams = Fentanyl 10 micrograms
NR = not recommended
When switching from one opioid to another, reduce the dose by 25% to 50% with adequate breakthrough medication
When switching to methadone, reduce the equianalgesic dose by 75% to 90%
Breakthrough medication should be available when controlled release medications are being used
All opioid medications should be carefully dosed and titrated with consideration for the individual patient and the medical condition of the patient

Sources: American Pain Society. (2008). *Principles of Analgesic Use in the Treatment of Acute Pain and Cancer Pain;* Fine, P., & Portnoy, R. (2007). *Opioid Analgesia;* Inturrisi, C., & Lipman, A. (2010). *Bonica's Management of Pain*, pp. 1174–1175; Smith, H., & McCleane, G. (2009). *Current Therapy in Pain.*
Used with permission of the author.

Index